SO YOU HAVE PROSTATE CANCER TOO!

A Medical Scientist with Prostate Cancer
Asks Questions, Finds Answers

Dr Brian J. Meade

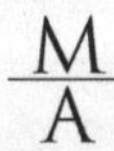
MICHELLE ANDERSON PUBLISHING
MELBOURNE

First published in Australia 2010
by Michelle Anderson Publishing Pty Ltd
P O Box 6032 Chapel Street North
South Yarra 3141 Melbourne Australia
Email: mapubl@bigpond.net.au
Tel: 03 9826 9028
www.michelleandersonpublishing.com

Cover design: Luke Harris, Chameleon Print Design
Typeset by: Midland Typesetters, Australia
Printed and bound in Australia by Griffin Press, Adelaide

National Library of Australia cataloguing-in-publication data

Author: Meade, Brian

Title: So you have prostate cancer too : a medical scientist with prostate cancer asks questions, finds answers / Brian Meade.

ISBN: 9780855723989 (pbk.)

Subjects: Prostate—Cancer.
Prostate—Cancer—Treatment.

Dewey Number: 616.99463

Disclaimer:
Although every effort was made to provide current reliable information based on scientific data, the author and publishers accept no liability for any errors or omissions which may be present in this book, and no liability is accepted arising directly or indirectly as a result of reading or other use of this book. If the reader has any doubts about the recommendations made here, medical or other appropriate health consultation is advised.

Dedicated to the men who have been – or may be – diagnosed with the condition, and to their 'support persons'

'So you have prostate cancer!' is Dr Brian Meade's personal encounter with a capricious common cancer through the strategy of integrative medicine and the mind of a scientist. In the past century the practice of non-mainstream medicine has been somewhat shunned by a hostile conservative medical profession, but in recent times there has been a more expansive and sympathetic attitude as manifest in this book. In his well researched cancer journey, Brian Meade pays tribute to the caring support of two surgeons both graduates of Monash University, where the philosophical approach in its formative years was to think broadly and laterally. Donald Murphy, a high profile orthodox urologist, who is Brian's local surgeon, has contributed some interesting and open minded insights to the book. The other surgeon is Professor Avni Sali, Australia's guru on integrative medicine, who has been a powerful medical and perhaps spiritual advisor to the author. The author also emphasises another powerful force in the healing process and that is the loving support of his family and that includes the person who prepares the all important meals.

Written for the man with prostate cancer, the main message is that you can control prostate cancer through 'proactive surveillance'. In parts of the book the material is presented in a question-answer format. The author with the foresight of his scientific background, explains how he has embraced the essential tenets of integrative medicine. These can be summarised as an optimal natural sensible diet, nutritional supplements, exercise, mind-body medicine and meditation

This is of nostalgic interest to this writer who as an educator has promoted the acronym of NEAT as an essential life style component of health prevention and the therapy for all disease. This stands for Nutrition (optimal, natural, balanced), Exercise, Avoidance or reduction of toxins (alcohol, nicotine, social drugs, caffeine, sugar, salt) and Tranqillity including recreation.

The author offers the reader many mind catching aphorisms such as

- Discipline your mind and your emotions
- Let food be your medicine
- Remember that 'heart healthy' is also 'prostate healthy' and vice versa
- Find a wise guide
- Get what your body needs from simpler healthy food
- You don't need to have a six-pack abdomen but you do need to be lean and tough

'So you have prostate cancer too!' is an empowering book for men with prostate cancer with a reassuring message that you can certainly control your disease. It collates the science, knowledge, experience and wisdom of scholarly minds.

Professor John Murtagh AM
BSc, Bed(Melb), MBBS, MD, DipObst(RCOG), FRACGP

Dr Brian Meade has prostate cancer, it is true, but he is determined to conquer it and I am pleased to be part of the medical team he has chosen for this venture. This book spells out his determination loud and clear; it is written with empathy, a sound knowledge base, and I think perhaps importantly, with optimism and humour.

Dr Anil Kaippilly Ebrahimkutty
MBBS, MD, MRCP, MRCGP, FRACGP
Senior General Practitioner, Tristar Medical Group,
Geelong, Victoria.

Prostate cancer is the most common cancer in men, excluding skin cancers. Throughout most of the Westernised world it is known that the first generation offspring (and beyond) of males who have emigrated from countries with low incidence of prostate cancer – such as Japan – to a country such as Australia, develop prostate cancer in accordance with the average incidence of the new country of residence. This epidemiological evidence demonstrates that the key factors leading to the development of prostate cancer are lifestyle and dietary factors, not genetic factors.

It has been the utilisation of this important data that has led to clinical research, which shows that it is also possible to influence the progression of this cancer by modifying lifestyle and dietary factors. It is of interest that these changes in lifestyle and dietary factors can actually improve genetic function.

Brian Meade decided to become an active participant in the treatment of his prostate cancer. Being a physiologist and educator, it was appealing to Brian that medical science supported his approach.

He set about elucidating the scientific information available on the care of men with prostate cancer, and discussing his personal experience with me and other colleagues in applying this information. He also offers insight into the difficulties experienced by the spouse in dealing with her partner's prostate cancer.

The final result of Brian's journey as a prostate cancer patient is a highly informative book, based on the best science. It is easy to read, containing lots of very useful, practical information. Though there are a number of books out there for the public about prostate cancer, I have not seen any as comprehensive as this text.

It is invaluable for men with prostate cancer to know that they can make changes to lifestyle and diet that have the power to actually influence the cancer. This book can show them how to do that.

Professor Avni Sali
MBBS, PhD, FRACS, FACS, FACNEM
Director – National Institute of Integrative Medicine
President – Australasian Integrative Medicine Association
International Council of Integrative Medicine

Acknowledgements

To the extent that the present work is accurate, authoritative and therefore valuable, the writer wishes to acknowledge the enormous debt he owes to Professor Avni Sali, Director of the National Institute of Integrative Medicine based in Melbourne. Although a top surgeon, Avni's first love was always Complementary Medicine. When it comes to Mind-Body Medicine and the impact of lifestyle on health, here indeed is a guru.

Not only has Professor Sali dramatically helped the writer to control his own prostate cancer, but he has been the inspiration behind this book. I never dreamt, after decades of watching him 'blaze a trail' in the areas of nutrition and natural medicine – and occasionally being fortunate enough to play a part – that he would be there as a friend and expert in my time of need. It was with his encouragement that I undertook to write the present work.

Thank you, Professor Sali.

My urologist, Donald Murphy MD, FRACS, stepped into a sudden breach and saved my only kidney. The other was removed when I was twenty, so I have grown attached to the one I have. Donald did not stop there, however. Although a senior urologist doing high-end research with the Royal

Australasian College of Surgeons, and although surgery is his primary *modus operandi*, he entered effortlessly into and supported therapeutic nutrition, supplements and lifestyle which constituted my wife's and my preferred path.

We think of Donald now as my urologist certainly, but more as research colleague and friend. We are very grateful for his endorsement of this book.

Dr Graham Lyons has been helping me with this book for a couple of years without ever realising it. Frequently I would email Graham if he wasn't in China or Indonesia or some other place out-of-town lecturing or solving their nutritional needs, and ask him a difficult question about supplements and prostate cancer. Inevitably a fact-filled reply would set me straight, complete with references.

Just yesterday he sent me an email asking, 'Did I ever send you this chapter which I wrote in that text-book?' It was great material on Nutritional Risk Reduction and Control of Prostate Cancer. I hope he doesn't send me any more till the book is published.

Graham has produced a concise document called Diet and Prostate Cancer. It over-views relevant cancer studies in terms of laboratory research, epidemiology and formal trials. It also deals with herbs, vitamins and other nutrients with strong scientific underpinning for the prevention and treatment of the condition. It is an excellent resource and is available free from Dr Lyons (see his address on back cover).

I must acknowledge the dedicated and enthusiastic contribution of my wife, Elizabeth. She had been a nurse, so she could enter into and discuss with me, the technical aspects of prostate cancer. She is a great cook, so that became a plus when we adopted a prostate-healthy diet. Above all, she is a wonderful soul-mate in the deepest sense of the word. And she laughs at all my jokes.

Our five sons have shown considerable interest in the book for some reason or other, and our daughters have been heard whispering things like epigallocatechin-3-gallate* into their husbands' ears.

It goes without saying, but I shall say it anyway, that this book would not have been published without the publisher. Michelle Anderson has shown remarkable patience during the frenetic last days of trying to interpret my multi-coloured drafts. Her advice has always been well-founded, no doubt because she has published many medically oriented books. I demurred only once on some suggestion or other and she graciously agreed.

It has become conventional to admit that any errors or other faults are entirely the property of the writer. I will follow the convention.

*Green tea extract.

Contents

Acknowledgements		vii
Foreword		xii
Chapter 1	Background and Structure of the book	1
Chapter 2	Active Surveillance	11
Chapter 3	Mind-Body Medicine	20
Chapter 4	Nutrition	37
Chapter 5	Supplements	66
Chapter 6	Exercise	89
Chapter 7	Treatment Options And New Initiatives	96
Appendix 1	Further thoughts on prostate cancer Mr Donald Murphy	117
Appendix 2	The support person's perspective Elizabeth Meade	122
Appendix 3	Notes for the advanced reader	126
Glossary of terms		147
References		161
Recommended Reading		175

Foreword

This treatise by medical research scientist Dr Brian Meade together with his wife Elizabeth, has been a journey of personal development for them both, as they have assessed and faced the impact of Brian's prostate cancer diagnosis on their lives.

Brian, a fit, vital and healthy man was diagnosed with prostate cancer at 74 years of age. This diagnosis is and was a challenge to his mortality; which has resulted in this research work, as they together sought to develop a contingent plan of action for his medical care.

General Norman H. Schwarzkopf Jnr. of Desert Storm fame, was diagnosed with prostate cancer in 1993, (PSA normal at 1.8 and abnormal prostate on DRE) when aged 59 years of age. He had a radical prostatectomy as treatment, which was successful according to Time Magazine, April 1996.

He is quoted as saying, "For me it was like war, the first thing you do is learn about your enemy and then you plan the battle".

So it has been for this couple. With Brian's research expertise they have assembled their plan of action, which is now shared through this book with others who are also in search of greater knowledge and the treatment possibilities for prostate cancer.

Pro-active surveillance as described in this book is an extension of care which is applicable to many prostate cancer patients.

Mr Donald Murphy
MD (Melb), MBBS (Mon), FRACS.
Senior Urologist – Geelong,
Medical Director – VTEC Skills Laboratory,
RACS Melbourne.

1

Background and Structure of the book

Q. Who wrote this book?

A. The writer of this book is a semi-retired Senior Research Fellow with the National Institute of Integrative Medicine. He was diagnosed at the age of 74 years with prostate cancer but decided, in consultation with his medical advisors, not to embark on the conventional primary therapies. Rather, he chose to go with 'pro-active surveillance' which will be described and explored later. His condition is now stable and his Prostate Specific Antigen, the main blood marker of prostate cancer status, is fine. Whether you have had treatment or not, 'active surveillance' can help you. The writer offers in this book, not so much his own opinions, but mostly those of the medical authorities and researchers extensively quoted and referenced.

Q. For whom was this book written?

A. This book is intended for men who have been diagnosed with prostate cancer. From autopsies, it is apparent that in the UK, about *half of all men* in their fifties have evidence

---

*There is a Glossary of technical terms at the back of the book for the keen reader, and Appendix 3 contains technical information for those even more advanced.

of cancer in their prostate, which rises to 80% by age 80, though only 3.8% will die from it! (Cancer Research UK: Prostate Cancer Incidence and Statistics, November 2008). The chances of actually being diagnosed are much less, which implies that not only will most men die *with*, not *from* the condition, but also that all men will get PC if they live long enough!

The book should also help men to avoid or reduce their chances of getting the disease. Prostate cancer is unusual in that there is NO CONSENSUS among doctors about the best treatment — or even whether any type of treatment at all is absolutely necessary (Johns Hopkins University Health Alerts, 19/12/2008. Emphasis is theirs). Note: Johns Hopkins has been ranked #1 of America's Best Hospitals for 18 consecutive years!

It is assumed that you, the patient, are under medical supervision – that is to say, you have a GP, a urologist and possibly a cancer specialist. A naturopath is highly desirable also, unless your GP or specialist is competent in complementary or integrative medicine – that is, medicine which takes a 'holistic' approach to health and disease, incorporating mind-body interaction, nutrition and life-style in general as fundamental factors in well-being.

When you were diagnosed with prostate cancer (PC), your doctor would have explained the nature and extent of your disease and the options available to you. He/she would have addressed the questions of how much your prostate cancer might threaten your life, how your age and other health conditions might affect your decisions, what treatments you can have and the good and bad points of each. With help and guidance from your medical team, you will have chosen either to embark on immediate surgery or a form of radiation, or possibly one of the forms of hormone therapy available, or to continue a wait-and-watch or Active Surveillance programme.

While this book is directed at men who have been diagnosed with prostate cancer, others who have not been diagnosed may find it useful. Specifically, men with first degree relatives who have the condition will be keen to take steps to prevent it*. The term 'proactive surveillance' is not usually taken in this sense, but it is certainly appropriate for *anyone* prepared to modify his lifestyle as the book recommends. As you will see, this offers potentially excellent preventive 'insurance' against the disease.

The book is pitched at the understanding of the ordinary reader. For those more medically informed, however, or for those who might like to have a deeper idea as to what's happening at the molecular level, more extensive information is offered in Appendix 3.

Q. What if I have already had treatment?

A. If you decided to have surgery or radiation, perhaps your doctor has also advised modification of lifestyle. This not only improves your chances against PC recurrence, but

---

*Regarding familial 'predisposition' to prostate cancer, it is commonly stated that having a first degree relative with the condition, doubles one's chances of getting prostate cancer. This is against the 'incidental' or general occurrence in the male population of about 10% (so-called sporadic gene abnormalities).

it considerably enhances your general well being including your immune and cardiovascular systems. Since no single therapy or combination of therapies can guarantee cure or 100% survival after any given number of years (Wilt, 2008), men who have undergone treatment may want to put in place some sort of insurance program against progression. There is very strong evidence (see later) that lifestyle modification is a good way to go if relapse is to be avoided.

Q. What if I decide to wait, or not to have therapy for whatever reason?

A. If you chose to wait before embarking on a particular intervention, various factors must be considered if you are not to miss the 'window of opportunity' for appropriate treatment. All of these issues are discussed in straightforward detail by the Australian Prostate Cancer Collaboration in their booklet, Localised Prostate Cancer, A Guide for Men and their Families. This is available – in Australia – from your urologist free of charge, or on loan.

Although this does not apply to the younger man with an aggressive form of the disease, prostate cancer is often more like a chronic condition of rather slow-growing nature. It is for the medical team to advise as to whether/ when immediate intervention 'with curative intent' is appropriate.

In this regard, it is worth mentioning a new study involving 200,000 men, which found that '. . . because of the excellent survival chances of older men diagnosed with early-stage prostate cancer with low-to moderate-grade tumors, (they) should not stop looking out for other illnesses . . .' (Goodwin et al., 2009). They found that the survival rate for such men was not substantially worse than men without prostate cancer. Their suggestion then, is that such men should focus on screening and prevention of cardiovascular disease and other cancers.

It is fortunate, of course, that a lifestyle which is good for PC is also good for all other ailments including cardiovascular disease. Improved nutrition is known to improve risk of heart disease, diabetes and obesity, and usually improves overall quality of life, increases energy levels, facilitates recovery and enhances the immune system (Ledesma, 2005).

In a recent trial in which subjects are randomly chosen either to receive a treatment or intervention, or to receive a placebo such as a 'sugar pill' (Ornish et al., 2005), men with confirmed prostate cancer were recruited to study the effects of comprehensive lifestyle changes on the progression of their disease. Prostate Specific Antigen or PSA levels decreased significantly in those undertaking the program. Essentially, it consisted of a vegan diet plus 'prostate-friendly' supplements (see Chapter 5), moderate aerobic exercise and stress management including meditation.

The Prostate Cancer Foundation was founded in 1993 to find better treatments and a cure for recurrent PC. It is now the world's leading philanthropic organisation for funding PC research. In the 2009 edition of their guide or 'White Paper' entitled *Nutrition, Exercise and Prostate Cancer*, one finds a fitting overview of the principles which form the basis of this chapter. Following is a brief excerpt from the Introduction:

Treatment options for prostate cancer are more effective than ever before. Yet, for many men, the diagnosis and treatment of cancer brings to their attention the need to change their diet and exercise behaviors. While the primary focus of the prostate cancer survivor is to live a life free of cancer, more men are beginning to realize that a healthy diet and regular exercise can be an important step toward preventing other diseases that commonly occur with aging, including heart disease and diabetes.

Exciting new data suggest that this same approach may also slow prostate cancer growth. This guide takes the best published evidence from population studies, basic science, and limited human studies, and puts them together in ways that make practical sense – with the overall goal of helping you achieve "thrivership" not just survivorship . . .

. . . most of our DNA is the software involved in determining how and when 30,000 genes are expressed. Regulation of this expression can be affected by environmental, nutritional, and other factors. These changes to the genome by external factors, called epigenetic changes, can have significant effects on a wide variety of molecular processes.

In fact, it is estimated that only 30% of processes normally associated with aging are dictated by genes, while 70% are under your personal control – through diet, exercise, and other lifestyle behaviors.

The Heart Foundation and The Cancer Council have made it clear that lifestyle – and particularly what we eat

– is critical in how we handle cardiovascular problems and cancer. A doctor who smokes cigarettes is an anachronism. So is a doctor who eats too much fat. And so is a doctor who is not interested in the relationship between nutrition and cancer. So choose your medical team wisely. See P29 for further information on Integrative Medicine.

Whether you have chosen to go for 'Active Surveillance' alone, or whether you chose a primary treatment but realise that active surveillance is still in your interests, you are now becoming 'pro-active' and this is your best chance to turn this into a manageable, chronic disease.

Overview and structure of the book.

Q. Could you give a summary of what the book is about and its structure?

A. A question-and-answer format with extensive references has been used in this work, since that ensures that the material expressed is not the brain-child of the author, but rather the accumulated knowledge of experts in the field of prostate cancer and related areas as they apply to Active Surveillance.

The attack on cancer seems to require a multi-pronged approach. This is not just because the causes are obscure, but also because individuals vary so much that any single therapy may work for one person and not so well for another. In Chapter 4 we will look at how cancer cells work and therefore what 'lifestyle' weapons – specifically nutrients – are needed against them. As a result of asking questions and pursuing answers from specialists and the most up-to-date medical journals and data bases, the following overall approach has emerged.

What is called 'Mind/Body Medicine' is the foundation on which the other lifestyle weapons are based. The reader might like to pursue the subject of mind-body medicine at the following web-site:

http://www.umm.edu/altmed/articles/mind-body-000355.htm.

A diagnosis of cancer is particularly stressful. This stress itself then initiates all sorts of psychological and pathological processes which make things much worse for the patient. A strong effort should therefore be made at the time of diagnosis, to offset this stress (Vitetta and Sali, 2008). In particular there arises a unique tension called 'PSA anxiety'. Awaiting the results of monthly or two-monthly or three-monthly tests can be worrisome and draining. We sometimes put too much focus on the PSA reading, however, and if it rises from 6.25 to 6.26 we get in a panic and can't wait till the next one comes in. A man who finds himself doing this should confide in his urologist or perhaps his GP, and seek further expert help. The expert will hopefully talk about Mind-Body Medicine and not simply prescribe anxiolytic drugs. I have found that meditation and vigorous exercise are excellent ways to deliver one from anxiety. You are especially blessed if you have a wise support person. See more in Chapter 3.

A study from Tel Aviv University found that stress plays a crucial role in cancer progression even if the primary tumour has been removed through operation (Ben-Eliyahu, 2007). This author and colleagues had previously demonstrated that stress adversely affects resistance to metastasis or spread of the cancer to other organs (Ben-Eliyahu et al., 2000).

In this context, it is well worth reading Ian Gawler's book, 'You can Conquer Cancer' (see Recommended Reading). Although it is of primary importance, mind-body medicine will be discussed later in the book because most cancer sufferers want to get straight into the 'nuts-and-bolts'. In other words, 'Is there something which I can begin straight away which should produce some early results?'

In terms of importance, after mind-body medicine comes nutrition. 'We are what we eat' isn't entirely true of course, but it says a lot. We absolutely need to be more aware of what to eat and what not to eat. Obesity is bad news for everybody, but 'caloric restriction' is strongly indicated for prostate cancer patients. And yet the nutritional program should be both interesting and fulfilling in every way. I can testify to my wife's imaginative cooking which is not just super-healthy, but tasty! And one should never be hungry.

Since we as cancer patients cannot eat all the specifics that the literature recommends, supplements become important. These may be in capsule, tablet or liquid form. But they need to be carefully controlled and once again the medical team is critical if we're not going to cause problems unwittingly.

Finally there is exercise. Not only does exercise keep your weight down, but as you will see it improves your immune and cardiovascular systems, it enhances your outlook on life and plays an absolutely vital role in PC prevention and treatment.

At the end of the book there is a glossary of terms, because many people who are reading this will not be familiar with biochemistry, endocrinology, physiology and pathology. Even one's urologist or other specialist may not be sensitive to this and may use technical terms which puzzle and even confuse the patient.

It is not necessary for a patient to understand scientific jargon, but it is a great help if he or his 'support person' can do so. Not only does this understanding help communication with the medical professionals, but it opens up a whole new and exciting world of atoms and molecules and the mind-boggling activities going on in the cells of the body. Even when an illness overtakes us, it can still be fascinating and indeed helpful to track what's happening, and at the very least to marvel at how fearfully and wonderfully we are made.

Let us explore what can be done in the way of lifestyle modification, why, and with what likely impact. Chapter 7 looks at Treatment Options and New Initiatives.

SUMMARY

The Take-Home Message is, you have considerable power to take charge of your cancer. Discover where this power lies and use it. It will be a worthwhile journey.

Whether you have chosen to go for 'Active Surveillance' alone, or whether you chose a primary treatment but realise that active surveillance is still in your interests, you are now becoming 'pro-active' and this is your best chance to turn this into a manageable, chronic disease.

2

Active Surveillance

Q. What exactly is 'active surveillance'?

A. Whereas 'watchful waiting' is simply monitoring the condition to see if it gets worse, active surveillance means that some strategy is in operation along with the monitoring. The monitoring in the latter case is usually also more vigorous. Other terms used for Active Surveillance are 'expectant management' or 'selective delayed intervention'. 'Pro-active surveillance' means that a much more aggressive offensive is mounted against the cancer than in conventional active surveillance, but still without any adverse 'harms' and in fact with many physical and psychological benefits.

Q. Among the experts, what is the current thinking on the usefulness of Active Surveillance in different situations?

A. Results of a 12-year study reported in the *Journal of the American Medical Association* showed only a 0.5% difference in the number of prostate cancer deaths between men treated with radiation therapy or radical prostatectomy and those whose cancers were managed with active surveillance (Johns Hopkins Health Alert 11th June 2009, 'Prostate Disorders: The Case for Active Surveillance').

Dr Lawrence Klotz, senior urologist at the University of Toronto Department of Urology, has written most extensively on this subject. In October 2008, he published an article in the World Journal of Urology in which he addresses the matter of potential 'over-treatment' (Klotz L, 2008a). He states that the contemporary screening for prostate cancer by means of Prostate Specific Antigen (PSA) measurement has resulted in the detection of prostate cancer (PC) in many men who are not destined to die from the disease.

One approach to reduce potential over-treatment, is to treat selectively by just observing patients with favourable risk disease, 'and treating only the subsets who are reclassified as higher risk over time, based on biochemical or pathological progression of disease'.

It is also the case that when primary intervention fails, many physicians recommend that rather than initiating immediate hormonal therapy for example, the patient might employ Active Surveillance, typically intervening only when PSA rises at a very rapid rate or to high levels or when clinical signs or symptoms of metastatic disease ensue (Saxe et al., 2005).

Urologists at Johns Hopkins have the policy not to treat patients who have a rising PSA as the only evidence of recurrent PC. At the heart of this approach is the realisation that men do not die of an increasing PSA, but of cancer metastatic to bone and other organs (Myers, 2007). In other words they use Active Surveillance until metastases are evident on medical examination or investigation.

Approximately one half of men diagnosed with low-risk prostate cancer undergo surgery or radiation therapy when active surveillance may have been a more appropriate initial response, according to a research team at the University of Michigan. Criteria for classification into the 'lower risk' PC group were men of any age with tumours which look normal under a microscope and are called well-differentiated, or men 70 years or older at diagnosis with tumours which look fairly normal under a microscope and which are called moderately-differentiated. Approximately one third of the 71,602 men in the reviewed group were classified as having lower risk PC and 55% of these underwent 'curative therapy' which equated with over-treatment (The Prostate Cancer Charity News story, 2007).

Dr Chris Parker, honorary consultant in clinical oncology at Royal Marsden Hospital in Surrey, England, was interviewed by Renal and Urology News in 2007. This was with regard to research reported in the Journal of the American Medical Association in 2006, indicating that treatment was preferable to surveillance. Asked the question, "When, if ever, is active surveillance the right choice for patients with prostate cancer?" Dr Parker replied, "I would turn the question around and ask, 'Given the lack of evidence from randomized trials in localized, screen-detected low- and intermediate-risk prostate cancer, when, if ever, is immediate treatment an appropriate strategy?'.

"Most men with screen-detected prostate cancer do not need treatment," he continued. "It is important to note that the JAMA study has a number of very important limitations. First, it was not randomized, so it's possible that any differences in outcome between the treatment groups relate to an imbalance in unknown but important prognostic factors. Second, the difference in overall mortality between the two groups was very small because a majority of deaths were from causes other than prostate cancer.

"Active surveillance is for men for whom it is uncertain whether or not aggressive treatment is necessary. The aim is to target treatment to those who need it, and avoid treatment in those who do not. So, when it comes to patient selection for Active Surveillance, we should identify men for whom delayed treatment, if it does become necessary, would be as effective as immediate treatment. We are not trying to identify only those men for whom treatment will never be needed. Men who will never need treatment don't need active surveillance.

"It is important to point out that the morbidity – unhealthy side-effects – of radical treatment for prostate cancer is well known. In my view, patients should weigh the known morbidity of treatment against the unknown potential for improved survival. If treatment had no morbidity, then treating all patients would make sense. At present, the morbidity of all radical treatment options remains significant, and active surveillance is therefore an attractive alternative. Ten years ago there were enough data to say that active surveillance makes sense as an approach to low-risk prostate cancer. Now we have data from Active Surveillance, with 10-year follow-up, demonstrating that the results are satisfactory.

"Ultimately, the choice between Active Surveillance and immediate treatment is a value judgment. The advantage of Active Surveillance is that most men will avoid the morbidity of treatment. The possible advantage of immediate treatment is that the patient might have better long-term survival. But this is not known. I have estimated that a 14-year treatment delay would probably increase prostate-cancer mortality just 7.5%. We'll have better data when the START (Standard Treatment Against Restricted Treatment) trial is completed. It is currently comparing these two approaches.

"Of course, when it comes to determining treatment, the patient's values are of paramount importance. Only the patient knows how important it is to him to avoid impotence or incontinence. And only the patient can trade off the risk of side effects against the potential for improved survival. The doctor's role is to provide the best available information so that the patient can make his judgment. If treatment had a 50% risk of impotence and a 2% improvement in 15-year overall survival, most men would choose not to have it."

Dr G. Lu-Yao and colleagues presented data to the American Society of Clinical Oncology in 2008, to demonstrate that after 10 years of Active Surveillance, prostate-specific mortality was 6%, 3% and 17% for low, moderate and high grade cancer in a population of 9,000 patients. They concluded that, since the majority of men with non-aggressive PC died of competing causes of death and did not develop complications that required surgery or radiation therapy, Active Surveillance may be a reasonable option for elderly patients with localized PC, especially among those without high-grade cancer.

Given all the above, it still needs to be emphasised that it is not the intention of this book to influence one's decision about treatment options. The primary focus is on Active Surveillance – or more exactly, pro-active surveillance

– though it is certainly hoped that the above supports its value in prevention, and as adjunct in the case of the diagnosed patient whether he chooses therapy or not.

Q. What is involved in the approach to Active Surveillance used by Dr Klotz?

A. In 2005, Dr Klotz set out the conditions or parameters which are now commonly used for Active Surveillance (Klotz L, 2008b). Patients are followed every three months for the first 2 years and every 6 months thereafter. Serum PSA measurement and Digital Rectal Examination are done at each visit and repeat biopsy is performed at 18 months after study enrolment.

As mentioned above, there are other forms of Active Surveillance, however. That is to say, while the monitoring methods may be the same or similar, other non-invasive strategies may be in place as in the studies by Ornish and Saxe. These variants will be addressed in detail later.

Q. What sorts of results have been achieved with the Klotz approach?

A. The largest, most mature Phase 2 study of Active Surveillance has reported an 85% overall survival and 99% disease-specific survival, that is, only 1% died from PC. There was a follow-up period of approximately 8 years (range 2–11 years). It is to be noted that this form of Active Surveillance does not incorporate any lifestyle intervention, which after all is what this book is about.

In the above study, Klotz used what is called the 'number needed to treat' method to compare radical surgery of the prostate (radical prostatectomy) with Active Surveillance. Between 80 and 90 prostatectomies would need to be performed for each prostate cancer death (which would be) avoided in a 'favourable risk, screen-detected population'. This means that Active Surveillance of this kind is more successful than surgery.

Q. Which other experts support Active Surveillance?

A. Firstly, keep in mind that the question is not 'Primary therapy or Active Surveillance?' The two are not mutually exclusive and Active Surveillance after therapy makes real sense. Nevertheless, in line with the thinking mentioned above, more and more published articles demonstrate that many men with non-aggressive PC detected by PSA screening will not exhibit disease progression during their lifetime; their treatment and associated side effects are unnecessary (Etzioni, 2002; Ornish, 2005).

Miller et al., in 2006 argued that approximately one half of men diagnosed with low-risk prostate cancer undergo surgery or radiation therapy when watchful waiting (Active Surveillance) may have been a more appropriate initial response.

Leibovici et al., in 2006 drew a distinction between watchful waiting and Active Surveillance. Preliminary results show that more patients remain on Active Surveillance than on watchful waiting. They explain that Active Surveillance is a novel approach consisting of avoiding the risks of therapy, while allowing early detection of those who are prone to progress. In these high-risk individuals, delayed active treatment is offered.

Dall'Era and colleagues in 2008 reviewed the literature on Active Surveillance. 'It appears that a limited number of men on Active Surveillance have required treatment, with the majority of such men having good outcomes after delayed selective intervention for progressive disease.'

In September 2008, the Prostate Cancer Research Institute held a Conference in the US which was addressed by experts in oncology, urology and nutrition. A couple of excerpts only will be provided, but proceedings of the Conference are available on the Internet (see again under Ch 5, Supplements).

Report on the 2008 Prostate Cancer Conference – Los Angeles, California, September 6-7

> *Dr. Peter Carroll, MD is on the faculty of the Department of Urology at the University of California in San Francisco. His talk was titled "Monitoring Prostate Cancer Without Immediate Treatment." Dr Carroll stated that Active Surveillance can extend survival periods by 10 to 15 years.*
>
> *Charles "Snuffy" Myers, MD, medical oncologist from Earlysville, VA, speaking on 'An Aggressive approach to Metastatic Disease; Diagnosing and Treating Oligo-metastasis (limited metastasis)', introduced himself as someone who has been fighting his own advanced prostate cancer for more than 9 years.*
>
> *Spread of prostate cancer to lymph nodes and bone is generally very slow, he said, and a single bone metastasis can hold, without growing or spreading, for up to 10 years.*

Other medical reports on similar lines have been offered by Van As et al., (2007), Loblaw et al. (2007) and Barocas, (2006).

SUMMARY

The Take-Home Message is, get together a knowledgeable, pro-active team of advisors including someone skilled in holistic or complementary medicine.

There is a vast amount of scientific underpinning for the attitude, 'If I enter into this fight with the right advisors, whether I am about to embrace aggressive intervention, or whether I have done this already, the principles of Active Surveillance will give me my best shot at achieving my goals.'

3

Mind/Body Medicine

Meditation/Relaxation

It is more important to know what sort of person has a disease than to know what sort of disease a person has.
—Hippocrates

Q. What exactly is mind-body medicine?

A. There is vast literature on this. As a starting point, consider the powers of positive thinking and auto-suggestion. These phenomena are well known ('mind-over-matter'), and a good example might be the so-called 'placebo effect'. This means that a person given an inactive substance but believing it to be active, very often experiences the same effect as if it were in fact the active substance.

Given the profound relationship between the mind and the body, it has long been acknowledged that the state of one's mind will have an impact on the state of one's body for better or worse. Hippocrates also wrote, "Natural forces within us are the true healers of disease." And yet over recent centuries, we have begun to think that the body was indeed separate from the mind and anyone interested in treating physical illness by treating the mind was indulging in 'hocus-pocus' or virtually witchcraft.

Whereas contemporary western medicine tends to use an exclusively biologic-genetic model of health, recent research strongly supports the adoption of a 'biopsycho-social' paradigm. This general approach to mind-body medicine is succinctly explained by Astin et al., (2003). With specific regard to prostate cancer, Coker in 1999 wrote an excellent article on the integration of mind-body medicine with traditional methodologies and therapies.

In medicine, the way our mental state affects our immune system is also becoming clear (Antoni et al., 2006). The 'short-term' immune response actually prompts the immune system to action, but chronic stress seems to act differently and depresses the immune system especially in the sick and elderly. Evidence from both animal and human studies suggests that long-term stress weakens a person's immune system (Reiche et al., 2004). In general, stronger relationships have been found between psychological factors and cancer *growth* and *spread* than between psychological factors and cancer development.

Dr Charles Myers, the medical oncologist mentioned earlier, wrote a book called 'Beating Prostate Cancer: Hormonal Therapy and Diet' (see Recommended Reading). In this, he argues convincingly on the issue of mental attitude when it comes to cancer, pointing out that every doctor knows of patients who just 'gave up' and died, whereas others who maintained or developed an optimistic approach to their condition, survived.

Dr Ainslie Meares, a Melbourne psychiatrist, reported a number of cases of regression of cancer following intensive meditation (Meares, 1982) and, given the above research, it is likely that there is a connection with the immune system.

Dr Bruce Lipton is well known for his research and books on the 'biology of belief'. His revolutionary thinking addresses the way in which even our genes are under the control of our minds and also under the influence of minds other than our own! (Lipton, 2005).

The success achieved by the Alcoholics Anonymous program illustrates the power of the mind over a stressful and apparently intractable situation. So successful has this '12-step' program been, that there are now many groups of people with one form or another of addiction based on these principles. Amongst these are Cocaine Anonymous, Kleptomaniacs and Shoplifters Anonymous, Gamblers Anonymous, Methadone Anonymous, Overeaters Anonymous and Sexaholics Anonymous.

Hypnosis is a procedure well known for its therapeutic use, and it is fundamentally the action of mind over body. Amongst the conditions for which it has proven to be beneficial are the management of pain in dentistry, control of panic attacks, reduction in severity of asthma and some allergies, even the stabilization of blood sugar levels in diabetic patients.

The influence of psychosocial factors on cancer has been well studied. For example, Schussler et al., in 2001 reviewed clinical investigations dealing with the influence of such factors on human immunity. The literature is convincing that psychological/psychopathological factors can promote cancer.

Conversely, the literature is equally convincing that correcting such factors can control or even reverse cancer as indicated above. For the interested reader, there is a well researched connection between the endocrine or hormonal and the immune systems. The appropriate subject is called PsychoNeuroEndocrinology or PNE.

One important aspect of mind-body medicine is the recognition that we, the patients, need the assistance of others. To have a confidante is very important – someone who understands us at a very deep level and who cares for us. This will commonly be a spouse/partner/friend rather than a medical practitioner. An Australian study on ten year survival in aged Australians, found that older people with a large circle of friends were 22 percent less likely to die during the study period than those with fewer friends (Giles et al., 2005)

In 2008, Schnall and colleagues at the University of Virginia reported a remarkable effect of friendship on perception. In the Journal of Experimental Social Psychology (Vol. 44, pp 1246–1255) they described how a group of students was taken to the base of a steep hill preparatory to climbing it. The students were asked to estimate the steepness of the hill and the likely difficulty in climbing it. The participants were divided into two groups, some standing next to friends while others stood alone. The students who stood with friends gave lower estimates of the steepness of the hill, and the longer the friends had known each other, the less steep the hill appeared.

While it not intended in this book to go further into the matter of companionship, the role of pets is well worth thinking about and following up. Considerable research has established the very significant social and health benefits of the 'companion animals', especially dogs.

Q. The term meditation has religious overtones. Is that what is meant?

A. Perhaps the term 'mental relaxation' might be more accurate. That is not to say that religious meditation is inappropriate in the context of cancer therapy. Dr Ian Gawler in his book, 'You can conquer cancer' (see Recommended Reading) suggests the use of any 'mantra', spiritual or otherwise, which will achieve the depth of mental unwinding and calm necessary for this purpose. In fact he suggests that whereas some Christians might repeat the 'Ave Maria', people of other persuasions would likely have a different prayer or phrase. Non-believers may repeat any word or sound which is meaningful to them. Such a device in Transcendental Meditation is well known.

For those who do have a deep religious Faith, however, studies show that it is advantageous for them to lean on their understanding of, and hope in, a Creator who is concerned for their well-being. McCullough et al., did an analysis of 42 studies on this topic in 2000 and the results clearly indicate that religious observance leads to a longer and healthier life. Religious commitment was also linked to longer life and life satisfaction in research conducted by Clark and Lelkes, 2006.

Believing in God can help block anxiety and minimize stress, according to new University of Toronto research that shows distinct brain differences between believers and non-believers. This was reported in *Science Daily*, March 5th, 2009.

Possessing a greater purpose in life is associated with lower mortality rates among older adults according to a new study by researchers at Rush University Medical Center.

Patricia A. Boyle PhD, and her colleagues from the Rush Alzheimer's Disease Center, studied 1,238 community-dwelling elderly participants from two ongoing research studies, the Rush Memory and Aging Project and the Minority Aging Research Study. None had dementia. Data from baseline evaluations of purpose in life and up to five years of follow-up were used to test the hypothesis that greater purpose in life is associated with a reduced risk of mortality among community-dwelling older persons.

Purpose in life reflects the tendency to derive meaning from life's experiences and be focused and intentional, according to Boyle. After adjusting for age, sex, education and race, a higher purpose of life was associated with a substantially reduced risk of mortality. Thus, a person with high purpose in life was about half as likely to die over the follow-up period compared to a person with low purpose. (*Science Daily* June 18, 2009).

Q. How do I get my man to follow a meditation regime? He is a 'go-getter' and not easy to handle!

A. (by the author's wife!) My own husband is a Type-A personality plus plus plus! He has a very fertile imagination and lots of intellectual energy which needs harnessing. His relaxation or 'meditation' periods are therefore of critical importance. The morning and evening sessions are no problem – it's trying to get him to stop and unwind completely for a few minutes mid-morning and mid-afternoon which is the challenge. When he 'behaves himself', however, we can both see the results. He is calmer, more at ease and even more at peace.

We follow a system called progressive relaxation, which involves tensing the muscles for a few seconds and letting go. You start with your lower leg muscles and work your way up to the forehead. There are good books on the procedure. Because we are Christians, we use brief prayers as a mantra to gradually still the restless mind, but Muslims will use another method, Jews another and atheists will find yet another mantra which suits them.

Breathing is very important. Slow, rhythmic breathing is a time-honoured way of acquiring peace and tranquillity. The anxious person breathes rapidly in a 'fight-and-flight' or 'sympathetic' mode, sometimes to the point of hyperventilation, rapid pulse, raised blood pressure and so on. On the other hand, when we are breathing out in a slow and controlled manner, we bring the 'parasympathetic' or relaxation system into action. So if we can sit or lie quietly and breathe in calmly for, say, three seconds, then breathe out gently for, say, seven seconds, we are overriding the adrenalin response and the attendant anxiety.

The other good thing is that this form of breathing while counting or while murmuring some mantra or prayer, keeps our attention on the present moment. It does not take much effort to do this, and yet many of us wrestle unsuccessfully with fears or worries about the past or the future, trying by shear will-power to stop such thoughts. How much more pleasant, and more effective, to relax in the present which precludes unhappy excursions into the past and the future.

Spiritual writers all consider this resting in the present moment as *the* way to find the Transcendant (see References, Dr Tim Ewer).

Q. Can I teach myself to 'meditate'?

A. It is possible, and there are CDs available which can help. Nevertheless it is far, far better to have lessons in the art from an experienced teacher. And to become proficient in meditation at a level which will impact on your prostate cancer, daily practise is essential.

Q. I am concerned for my wife. My condition worries her although she tries not to show it. Is there anything I (or others) should be doing?

A. Get her involved. Share! As mentioned above, everyone needs a 'confidante' or someone whom they trust implicitly and in whom they can confide. Ideally this should be a spouse/partner/best friend but one can almost always find a 'support person'. A diagnosis of cancer is really a time for growth and mutual appreciation. Spend more 'quality time' together. Make plans. If you are 'believers', pray together. So long as you are each deeply concerned for the other, this journey will be a rewarding one and it will have profound therapeutic effects.

Support persons are too often neglected when illness strikes. A diagnosis of cancer in general – and, in the case of men, prostate cancer in particular – can have a dramatic impact on the patient and also on the support person.

The hope is that the clinician would handle the situation delicately, with compassion and with a positive approach. In the case of PC, the positive approach would surely outline some/most of the facts mentioned above and the most promising paths which can be taken.

While the information and advice has to be realistic, if well delivered it will be as encouraging as possible to the patient rather than leaving him (and the support person) in a state of shock and depression. Literature is helpful, but the clinician, taking into account the temperament of the patient which he/she should know well, will take whatever time is needed to inform and encourage the support person whose role is really critical. Such information and encouragement should be on-going.

Q. Since diagnosis, I have been anxious, depressed and can't sleep. I have been on medication but the side effects are almost as bad as the depression. My doctor more or less says to 'hang in there'! Now my wife is suffering too!

A. Meditation can help. Pay special attention to your breathing. Rhythmic, slow inspiration followed by slow, prolonged exhalation while relaxing all over – especially shoulders and forehead (see P26).

Good aerobic exercise will also help as does sunlight! Diet-wise, perhaps including sardines, cherries, walnuts and bananas would help. These increase your intake of either serotonin or tryptophan – ask your doctor to explain the rationale and to perhaps re-visit your medication.

With regard to sleep, this is a vital health issue. Sound and adequate sleep is mandatory for absolutely everyone, and you must do whatever is required to achieve this. Meditation will help, but you will probably require medical input for advice on appropriate herbs or even medications on a temporary basis. See also next question.

Q. I'm not completely confident in my medical advisor (GP or perhaps urologist or other). Can/should I look elsewhere?

A. First, give him/her every chance. Say that you are a little concerned and you feel that perhaps you are too demanding. If still not satisfied that the doctor has enough time/concern/knowledge, ask for a second opinion. No good doctor will object.

Always seek the advice of a doctor qualified in Integrative Medicine. Such practitioners are available world-wide, and the following sites should be helpful: www.aima.net.au and also www.acnem.org

Q. What is the connection between stress and health?

A. There is a huge literature addressing this question. An excellent overview of the subject has been offered by Professor Dean Ornish in his 'Spectrum Program'. In his on-line Preventive Medicine Research Institute site, he begins with the following basic explanation:

'Stress can be defined as the response of the human organism to any change or demand. Whether the demand or stress is positive or negative, the body responds automatically. The stress response is coordinated in the body by a part of the nervous system called the autonomic – or automatic – nervous system. This system has two divisions, the sympathetic and the parasympathetic nervous systems. The sympathetic nervous system controls the stress response and the parasympathetic nervous system controls the opposite or relaxation response.

When you experience a life change or demand, the sympathetic nervous system sends messages to muscles, organs and glands, which help the body react. Powerful chemicals like adrenaline, cortisol and aldosterone, and other neurotransmitters released by the adrenal glands and other organs, have multiple effects on the body.'

He then proceeds to list various functions which are affected by stress such as heart rate, muscle tension, increased blood sugar, rapid breathing and so on. A little further on he comes to the point in question – stress and health. He writes,

'These effects are adaptive in the short term and help a person prepare for dealing with the stress. When stress is chronic, these physical reactions can lead to disease. For a person with coronary heart disease, for example, some of these effects can lead to chest pain, shortness of breath, palpitations and coronary artery spasm and sudden blockages of coronary arteries (i.e., angina, irregular heartbeats or a heart attack). Other stress-related illnesses can include insomnia, sexual dysfunction, hyperactivity, ulcers, chronic headaches, backaches and high blood pressure.

'Aside from the physical effects, there are psychological and mental reactions to stress (such as) anxiety, depression, anger, irritability, decreased concentration and memory.' Ornish concludes this section by discussing the para-sympathetic system in some detail, emphasising that it brings about a relaxation response in the body. He mentions decreased blood pressure, decreased heart rate, decreased rate of breathing, feelings of calm and tranquility, and a healthy immune system.

Professor Avni Sali and colleagues in Australia have explored the effects of stress on health and the ramifications relating to cancer amongst other pathologies. A review of mind/body interactions – which involve hormones, neurotransmitters, neuropeptides and cytokines – was published by these researchers in 2005. They conclude that the advances in mind-body medicine research together with healthy nutrition and lifestyle choices can have a significant impact on health maintenance and disease prevention.

Professor Sali is currently involved in writing a text-book entitled *A Guide to Evidence Based Integrative and Complementary Medicine* (Elsevier, authors Kotsirilos V, Vitetta V, Sali A.) to be published in May 2010. He has written the chapter on cancer, and the work will be an excellent reference for nutrition and Mind-Body medicine.

Perhaps all of the above can be summed up in the commonly quoted equation,

Genotype + lifestyle = phenotype.

Genotype refers to the genetic composition of our cells, whereas phenotype means the way the genotype is actually expressed, or how we actually look.

Let us now look at the way in which stress affects our immune system, because therein lies a major key to this question.

Q. So what exactly is the relationship between mind/body, the immune system and cancer?

A. Recent research makes it clear that there is an association between psychological and behavioral factors and the incidence and progression of cancer. Kiecolt-Glaser et al., published an illuminating review on this matter in 2002. They suggested that it is through the impact these behavioral and psychological factors have on the cellular immune response, including natural killer (NK) cell function, that they may ultimately affect the occurrence and progression of certain tumors.

They began with a brief overview of the evidence that PsychoNeuroImmunology (PNI) research with healthy individuals may be relevant to cancer. They then linked extant PNI research findings with tumorigenesis – development of a tumor – and drew upon two important PNI findings relating psychological distress to two important aspects of carcinogenesis: (i) poorer repair of damaged cellular DNA and (ii) modulation of apoptosis or cell suicide. Finally they focus on the implications of intervention research in cancer patients for cancer progression and treatment.

Before reviewing the evidence regarding stress-related immunological changes, they noted that one recurrent concern in the literature is the question of the significance of the immune system for cancer. Cancer is comprised of a heterogeneous group of diseases with multiple etiologies, and immunological involvement varies across different cancers. Those cancers that are induced by chemical carcinogens – e.g. lung cancer – may be less influenced by psychological, behavioral and immunological factors than cancers that are associated with a virus, which tend to be immunogenic. Suppression of cellular immunity is associated with a higher incidence of certain types of tumors. See Appendix 3 for further information.

Additionally, some researchers have questioned whether stress-related immune changes are of either the type or the magnitude to influence tumor growth and metastases. While such issues were beyond the scope of their paper, they state that compelling evidence exists for the role of cells, such as Natural Killer (NK) cells, in resisting the progression and metastatic spread of tumors once they have developed.

Surprisingly, macrophages – pathogen destroyers in the blood which are part of our immune surveillance – have on their cell membranes receptors for endorphins or 'mood-enhancers'. This suggests that macrophages may be influenced by mood and is consistent with the observed relationship between mind-state and immunity.

In 2007, Academic Press published a most comprehensive book called *Psychoneuroimmunology* which was edited by Robert Ader. He is a professor at the University of Rochester and it was he who first promoted the idea of PNI in 1975. He is highly credentialed and a prolific author on this subject. PNI is the study of interactions among behavioural, neural and endocrine, and immunologic processes of adaptation, and the contributors are world experts in the related disciplines. The sorts of topics covered in this book are mainly for the keener reader and include:

Immune responses, Integrative immunology, Adrenergic regulation of immunity, Emerging concepts for the pathogenesis of chronic inflammatory diseases, Cross-talk or interaction among IGFs.

Further recent research on mind-body-medicine.

A group of researchers at UCLA recently used high-resolution magnetic resonance imaging (MRI) to scan the brains of people who meditate. In a study published in the journal *NeuroImage*, the researchers report that in the brains of long-term meditators there were significantly larger volumes of the hippocampus and areas within the orbito-frontal cortex, the thalamus and the inferior temporal gyrus – all regions known for regulating emotions.

Research has confirmed the beneficial aspects of meditation. In addition to having better focus and control over their emotions, many people who meditate regularly have reduced levels of stress and bolstered immune systems.

There were no regions where controls had significantly larger volumes or more gray matter than meditators. Because these areas of the brain are closely linked to emotion, these might be the neuronal underpinnings that give meditators the outstanding ability to regulate their emotions and allow for well-adjusted responses to whatever life throws their way. (Reported in *Science Daily*, May 13th 2009)

Q. What then is PsychoNeuroEndocrinology?

A. PsychoNeuroEndocrinology or PNE, is the clinical study of hormonal fluctuations and how they impact on behaviour (and therefore health). Since endocrine disorders lead to illness, and since it is postulated that the state of one's mind can influence the endocrine system, PNE becomes important in the pathophysiology (initiation and development of disease) of certain illnesses. It has recently been further postulated that cancer is one of those illnesses.

Linda Carlson and Sheila Garland reviewed the state of

the science in 2007. They cover such matters as psychosocial factors and disease initiation and progression, psychosocial intervention and survival, psychosocial interventions and immune/endocrine outcomes. They also address the broad array of study designs, samples, interventions and outcome measures involved. Of particular interest in our context is the section entitled 'Endocrine/Immune Measures and Disease Progression/Survival.'

Other areas of interest in the article relate to disease and hormonal factors like the role of oestrogen, testosterone, melatonin, growth factors and angiogenesis. The authors conclude that a comprehensive biopsychosocial model of disease progression will help to guide future research into PNE.

So while this is an oversimplification of a complex matter, the state of one's mind profoundly influences the state of one's body which includes one's health. If disease occurs as a result of stress, the pathways by which this happens are basically a) depression of the immune system and b) disturbance of the endocrine system. The aim of this chapter has been to high-light some of the major factors involved in mind/body medicine, and specifically to show how they can be controlled. Modifying one's attitudes and making the other lifestyle changes suggested in this book are important, and meditation not only facilitates these, but also has a major therapeutic value in PC.

The reader is strongly advised to visit (or hopefully re-visit) the University of Maryland web site below, to obtain a comprehensive overview of Mind/Body Medicine.

http://www.umm.edu/altmed/articles/mind-body-000355.htm.

SUMMARY

The Take-Home Message is, study and realise the immense power of mind over matter.

If you are able, read the literature about the immune system, PsychoNeuroImmunology and PsychoNeuro-Endocrinology as described in this Chapter. But more importantly, discipline your mind and your emotions. Preferably find a wise Guide, read some of the inspiring books by the publisher of this work and elsewhere, and be surprised at how your future unfolds.

4

Nutrition

"Let food be your medicine and medicine be your food."
—Hippocrates.

Experts now estimate that up to 90% of cancer of the prostate may have a dietary link (Johns Hopkins Special Report #2. Diet and Prostate Health, 2008) Before embarking on the Q&A segment, consider three interesting case studies of men diagnosed with PC at an early age.

Dr Charles Myers is an American medical oncologist who was diagnosed with prostate cancer in 1998 at the age of 55. He underwent aggressive therapies which halted progression. Well aware of the danger of relapse and progression, he began a program of vegetarian nutrition and various supplements. He now shares his insights into the disease via The Prostate Forum on-line.

In the year 2000, he addressed a sell-out audience in Sydney, a report of which was produced by the Prostate Cancer Foundation of Australia. Summing up his address, he argued that diet is at least as important as any other treatment for PC, and in his experience, a vegan/vegetarian diet can halve the rate at which PSA doubles, even for those on Active Surveillance.

Dr Myers has recently written two books on the value of nutrition in PC (see Recommended Reading). Myers says there is strong evidence from randomised trials that diet is a significant factor in the development of PC. He also believes that there is much stronger evidence for the benefit of changing diet than there is supporting radical prostatectomy or radiotherapy as effective treatments for the disease. 'In many ways,' he says, 'what you eat and what vitamins you take can have as much influence on creating a curative program as hormonal therapy or whatever treatment or combined treatments you choose.' (Beating Prostate Cancer: Hormonal Therapy and Diet p123).

Thomas Mueller, a 45-year-old attorney, learned in 2001 that he had PC. He decided that the potential side effects of the primary therapies were to be avoided at his age, and so he set about a rigorous program of nutrition and exercise. His PSA dropped from 4.0 down to 1.5ng/ml, an encouraging sign that his cancer was being held in check. His diet was particularly restrictive, consisting mainly of whole grains and vegetables. He avoided processed foods and sugars, fats, meat and dairy foods.

Although Mueller's approach may not appeal to everyone, he has achieved remarkable results. A repeat biopsy has revealed less extensive disease and his PSA has stayed low and stable. High resolution rectal imaging has found no evidence of cancer progression.

Thomas's rationale for taking on this approach, is that less toxic treatments will eventually arrive because of the pace of advancing medical technology and research. This will be referred to again in the segment on Insulin (Scholtz, 2006)

Mike Milken. The convicted Junk-Bond Wizard of the 1980s, when paroled, was diagnosed with PC in his forties with Digital Rectal Examination clearly indicating spread beyond the prostate capsule. He had a PSA of 24ng/ml, Gleason score 9 and metastases to the lymph nodes – in other words he was in a bad way. Mike immediately embarked on hormonal therapy which is common for men with advanced metastatic PC. Typically he responded to the androgen ablation, but knowing that relapse was quite likely he decided to take no risks at his age. He went onto a strict diet similar to that of Mueller's, and now, some years later, his cancer is under control. Mike's story is available on the Internet. He has become a major benefactor supporting prostate cancer research through American Nobel Laureate, Leroy Hood.

Q. It's hard to believe that our food can have much impact on cancer, isn't it?

A. Let's first look in a basic manner at how cancer works. Cancer results when cells accumulate errors in the genes – called genetic mutations – and multiply wildly. Normal cells differ from cancer cells in two main ways: the way they 'look' through a powerful microscope, and the way they behave. How they 'look' refers to the degree of 'differentiation' or the extent to which they appear like normal cells through a microscope. 'Well differentiated' cells look pretty much like normal ones. How they behave refers to how fast they grow, to what extent they 'invade' normal surrounding tissues, and whether they spread to other places like bone or lung or liver.

The enthusiastic reader who wants to acquire much more detail about prostate cancer cells, might search

Google for names like Donald Coffey, a world authority on the nuclear architecture of the diseased cells.

Any attack on PC therefore needs to address these issues. Diverse biological factors are involved as we will now show, but fortunately all of these lend themselves to 'phyto-therapy' (plant or herbal therapy) to a greater or lesser extent (Sali A, 2006; Ledesma N, 2005). The factors involved in the development of cancer are:

Hormonal balance

The male and female hormones both have a role in PC. Androgens – male hormones such as testosterone (T), dihydrotestosterone (DHT) and dehydroepiandrosterone (DHEA) – need to be in balance and they have to be in balance with the female hormones (oestrogens) which men also produce. These male oestrogens are generated in smaller quantities than they are in women of course. Then the oestrogens – given the abbreviation E because of the American spelling – need to be in balance themselves and the various forms of the oestrogens have to be in the right proportions as well.

Fortunately, many phytochemicals can help to re-establish and maintain the correct ratios for all of the above. Genistein from soy is a special example and will be mentioned again later. Diindolylmethane from broccoli sprouts is another.

Cell signalling

For cells to become active, for example in producing certain compounds for which they are specific such as insulin or adrenalin, they need to be stimulated in some way. Cell signalling may be via chemicals produced by adjacent or nearby cells, or it may be via hormones travelling round in the blood. Some signals excite cell responses, other signals dampen them down.

Once again, compounds from certain plants can impact on these signals. An example would be lycopene, which has been shown to negatively influence a 'survival' factor in cancer known as IGF-1 which will be discussed later. Saw palmetto and curcumin are other examples.

Cell cycle regulation

When a cell divides, it goes through well-defined stages from resting through various stages until the original cell splits into two 'daughter' cells. Cancer cells need to be stopped from uncontrolled dividing, and there are various nutrients which can help. An example of this is a chemical called indole-3-carbinol which is present in various vegetables such as cabbage, which can cause cycle arrest in PC cells.

Cell survival

Normal cells do not go on dividing forever. After a certain period or number of divisions, a cell stops dividing and dies. This natural cell death is called apoptosis. There are different ways this can occur, and phytotherapy can induce apoptosis. A chemical in green tea known as EpiGalloCatechin Gallate or EGCG is a well-known inducer of this anti-survival process in PC cells.

Cell differentiation

As indicated above, cell differentiation refers to the normal changes which equip the cell to do certain specific functions. Poorly differentiated cancer cells not only look strange under the microscope, but they also distort the tissue of which they are a part so that its 'architecture' also looks strange and unlike normal tissue.

Some phytochemicals can help to stimulate normal differentiation in cells which have been damaged and which are becoming cancerous. Vitamin D also does this.

Angiogenesis

Cancer cells need blood flow to bring nutrients and get rid of waste products, but because they are usually clumped tightly together they cannot access the normal capillaries which supply the normal tissue. So they themselves stimulate the production of new blood vessels called angiogenesis. They do this largely by stimulating the production of a protein called VEGF or Vascular Endothelial Growth Factor.

Quite a few nutritional supplements can inhibit VEGF and thus disadvantage the growing tumour. A good example is silibinin from milk thistle.

Metabolism of potential carcinogens

The liver produces chemicals whose job is to 'detoxify' impurities. What are called Phase 11 enzymes are particularly involved in this, and some phytonutrients stimulate the liver to produce these enzymes. Sulforaphane from broccoli sprouts is especially effective in this process.

Q. But what evidence is there that what we eat can cause or promote cancer?

A. Renowned US medical oncologist specialising in prostate cancer, Dr Stephen Strum, recently reviewed and critiqued a thorough and well-referenced article called

'Eating your way to prostate cancer' by William Falloon (on-line Life Extension Magazine Feb. 2007). The salient points can be summarised thus:

Prostate cancer cells are present in most men, yet only one in six men is ever diagnosed with the disease. Natural barriers help to protect some men from developing clinically diagnosable prostate cancer.

Poor dietary choices can break down the body's innate defences against the development of prostate cancer, while fueling its proliferation and spread. Consuming a healthy diet and specific protective nutrients can provide significant support against prostate cancer.

Here are some further points which Dr Strum makes in the February 2008 edition (v 11.1) of Insights from the Prostate Cancer Research Institute:

"PC PREVENTION: What we should have learned about PC in the last 10 years."

Many peer-reviewed publications show that specific dietary and life style changes as well as the usage of certain vitamins and supplements will reduce the incidence and/or the aggressiveness of PC. Fundamental to these findings is the basic concept that inflammation and its associated biological processes go hand-in-hand with all malignancies; PC is no exception. The inflammatory process involves the oldest hormonal system – the eicosanoid pathways. This hormonal system is found within the cell membrane of all cells.

"The production of what are termed 'bad eicosanoids' is significantly affected by the quantity and quality of the foods we eat – especially insulin-stimulating carbohydrates

– and whether or not we have a healthy intake of omega-3 fatty acids. If this metabolic road of bad eicosanoids is chosen, it is a bad detour since it increases the level of pro-inflammatory cytokines, tumor growth factors and activation of lines of communication (signal transduction pathways) that turn on tumor cell growth, invasion, angiogenesis and metastases.

"A basic knowledge of these facts leads us to understand the vital importance of the fuel we use to feed our cells – whether they are normal cells or malignant ones. Most of the civilized world is cognizant of the use of proper fuel to run machines such as automobiles and airplanes, but we ignore the very same concept in regard to the human machine."

The American Institute for Cancer Research (AICR) is the cancer charity that fosters research on the relationship of nutrition, physical activity and weight management to cancer risk, AICR's expert report (2008) recommends that cancer survivors receive nutrition advice from a health professional and follow AICR's guidelines to eat a mostly plant-based diet, get at least 30 minutes of physical activity a day and maintain a healthy body weight.

Q. How in fact do my eating habits affect my prostate cancer?

A. The old adage 'We are what we eat' has been validated more and more in recent times. Dr Charles Myers, the specialist in prostate cancer referred to above, in his book 'Eating Your Way to Better Health' (see later under

Recommended Reading), discussed the dietary components that appear to be involved in prostate cancer. Here are his main points:

There have been dramatic advances in our understanding of how dietary fat promotes the development of PC. We now know that components of dietary fat also stimulate and spread the growth of PC.

As cancers grow, they need to form new blood vessels to supply added food and oxygen. This process is called angiogenesis. A component of fat can dramatically enhance new blood vessel formation by PC cells. The immune response to cancer involves both natural killer cells and T cells that are also able to kill cancer cells.

PC cells can use dietary fat to produce chemicals capable of killing or disabling both of these immune cells. In summary, certain dietary fats allow the cancer cells to grow and survive, evade the immune system, and spread to other parts of the body.

Cancer cells do not move about in 'blind' fashion. They are able to sense the presence of other cells and tissues because these cells and tissues send out chemical messages. In the case of human prostate cancer cells, they are attracted to bone cells.

A particular fatty acid, Arachidonic Acid (AA) markedly stimulates the ability of human prostate cancer cells to move and invade. But it must first be converted to one of several powerful hormones. The family of hormones derived from arachidonic acid are called 'eicosanoids'.

Summary by Dr Myers:

Arachidonic acid is able to increase new blood vessel formation, enhance invasiveness, speed growth and block the death of prostate cancer cells.

Excess intake of essential omega-6-fatty acids increases the risk of disease or increases the severity of the disease. The evidence strongly suggests that one of these side effects might be metastatic prostate cancer.

Studies indicate that dietary fat did not influence the risk of localized prostate cancer, but did increase the risk of metastatic prostate cancer. When they examined specific foods, red meat, dairy fat, egg yolks, and creamy salad dressings emerged as significant risk factors for metastatic disease.

Dr Myers argues that if you switch to a vegan diet, you will significantly reduce arachidonic acid in your blood. Taking the additional step of switching to a low fat vegan diet, especially one that limits linoleic acid (precursor of AA), will reduce arachidonic acid levels to an even greater extent.

Myers also addressed the topic of nutrition and immunity in PC. 'In men over the age of 50, immune cells are common throughout the normal prostate tissue. If you examine radical prostatectomy specimens, you will find that immune cells are uncommon in prostate cancers of Gleason grades of 7 or higher. Some process has eliminated the immune cells from the higher-grade prostate cancers and the area immediately surrounding the cancer.

In 2002, Dr Myers did a presentation to the Sloan Kettering Medical Centre Prostate Cancer Support Group.

He quoted a study published in the Journal of Urology in 2001, in which a group of men who had rising PSA after prostatectomy, undertook a low fat 'heart-healthy' diet. The average PSA doubling time – that is, the time it takes for the PSA level to double – had been about six months, but this improved with the diet to eighteen months. Dr Myers stated that, 'By just taking on the diet and lifestyle change that would be good for heart disease, they effectively tripled their survival for prostate cancer.'

Another factor in the diet/PC story involves insulin. For many years there has been interest in Insulin-like Growth Factors (IGF, see p 49) and PC, but more recently, insulin itself has come into prominence. For example, in 2001, a study of Chinese men established that insulin levels may influence the risk of PC (Hsing et al., 2001). In 2005, a Swedish group showed that excess insulin is a risk factor for fatal PC (Hammarsten and Hogstedt, 2005).

In 2007, a Canadian group, building on the growing interest in dietary carbohydrate, fat intake and prostate cancer, postulated that high levels of insulin resulting from high intake of refined carbohydrates would lead to rapid growth of tumours. They found that indeed a diet high in refined carbohydrates is associated with increased tumor growth in mice (Venkateswaren et al., 2007).

Dr Michael Pollack, professor of oncology at McGill University led a study (2008) which found that men who are overweight and who have high insulin levels when they are diagnosed with prostate cancer may be more likely to die from the disease.

'I don't want to be sensationalist,' he said, 'but obesity effects and the insulin effects are so big that I think if you had to choose between being thin and having a low insulin level or having access to the best chemotherapy, you would be more likely to survive without chemotherapy.'

Food which is digested quickly causes a rapid and high insulin response. One of the roles of insulin is to facilitate the transfer of glucose into cells, though in fact the hormone has other less well-known functions. Stress hormones – such as cortisol and adrenalin – can also stimulate the release of insulin.

Dr Mark Scholz (2006) explains that, "Cancer cells divide rapidly and are therefore greedy for sugar, because it is necessary for their growth. This fact is dramatically illustrated by Positron Emission Tomography, or PET scan. The Pet scan uses radioactive sugar injected into the bloodstream to locate tumors throughout the body. PET can so effectively pinpoint growing, active groups of PC, that within a matter of minutes, the areas of high sugar uptake can be clearly seen in the scan images.

"Cancer cells require dramatically more glucose to survive and proliferate than normal cells. This is because cancer cells run on a primitive energy metabolism called anaerobic glycolysis that burns sugar without oxygen. Oxygen metabolism (aerobic glycolysis) allows the healthy cells of the body to extract many more molecules of energy from glucose than with anaerobic glycolysis.

"Diabetics – men with chronically high blood sugar – have less prostate cancer than normal men. How can we explain this? Diabetes is a disease of low insulin levels. We know that sugar in the blood is unable to enter the cells without the aid of insulin. Insulin is manufactured and stored in the pancreas until released into the blood in response to high glucose levels.

"The connection between diet and PC, therefore, appears to hinge only indirectly on blood sugar levels. It is not high blood sugar per se, but rather the high level of insulin, triggered by high blood sugars, that stimulates rapid PC growth. There are several reasons why this makes sense. Insulin is one of the most potent growth hormones in the body. Several studies have reported a connection between insulin and PC. Two of these studies show that high insulin levels, or a high sugar diet which causes high insulin levels, are connected with a higher incidence of PC. A third study has reported that increased insulin levels are associated with more high grade PC."

Barnard et al., in 2002 observed that insulin resistance – limited ability of insulin to act on cells – and compensatory hyperinsulinaemia or excess insulin in the blood, are thought to be the underlying factors in the metabolic or insulin-resistance syndrome and can be controlled by diet and exercise.

It is important now to understand a little more about Insulin-like Growth Factor (IGF) and its binding protein as they relate to PC. IGF-1 is a hormone very like insulin and is produced in the liver. There is strong interaction between IGF and various growth factors which are known to stimulate cell division.

Hormones produced by fat – especially belly fat – affect the ability of cells to properly take up insulin. This insulin resistance causes overproduction of insulin and IGF, both of which are potent stimulants for prostate cancer growth.

While there is some dispute as to the exact role of IGF in prostate cancer, there is considerable research into the compound, its receptor and insulin, and particularly into methods of enhancing the binding protein for IGF (IGF-BP). There has also been increasing evidence that insulin at physiological concentrations may play a clinically important role in breast cancer. Women with insulin levels in the top 25% of a particular study group had a doubled risk of recurrence and a tripled risk of death (Goodwin, 2008).

It has recently been found that an IGF/insulin receptor – that is, a protein in or on a cell membrane onto which a compound from the blood can lock – is present in all breast cancer subtypes and is related to poor survival (Law et al., 2008).

IGFs are capable of enhancing proliferation and inhibiting apoptosis in normal and malignant prostate cells, but IGFBP-3 is found to stimulate apoptosis (Vijayababu 2006).

Again, Wang and colleagues (2007) investigated the compound genistein (see later in Chapter 5) in its relation to PC. The rationale for their study was that the interaction between sex steroids and growth factor signalling pathways is thought to be critical in the development and differentiation of hormone-responsive tissues, and for cancer development in the prostate. In particular, the EGF- (Epidermal Growth Factor) and IGF-signalling pathways are involved in the regulation of cell growth and differentiation.

Estrogen action is strongly related to the EGF and IGF systems with evidence of interaction between them at several levels. Estrogen is another important player in the PC story (see Chapter 5, Supplements, DIM etc.).

With this background, it should be no surprise to find that excess insulin is bad news for PC sufferers. Swedish research urologists have established that excess insulin and other metabolic disorders precede deaths caused by prostate cancer. Hyperinsulinaemia, they concluded, is a promoter of clinical PC. Further, they suggest that insulin levels could be used as a marker of PC prognosis and tumour aggressiveness (Hammarsten et al., 2005).

Insulin has been further implicated in the development of PC. Insulin is known to increase cancer risk through its effect on cell proliferation, differentiation and apoptosis. In the last decade, converging evidence from epidemiological and clinical studies suggests that the insulin is involved in the development and growth of cancer of the prostate (Nandeesha, 2008).

Dr Strum, quoted above, has also commented further. "The only way to increase longevity is via caloric restriction. In the civilized world, especially the USA, there is an epidemic of diabetes mellitus that includes grade school children. The term adult onset diabetes mellitus (AODM) must be renamed because large numbers of children and teenagers are now being diagnosed with this type of diabetes, also called Type II diabetes mellitus.

"The factors that underlie the development of AODM are carbohydrate excess, caloric excess and a sedentary lifestyle. The same factors lead to cardiovascular disease and neurodegenerative disease.

"The typical diet in the Western world is overloaded with high glycemic foods – foods that stimulate insulin –

which in turn stimulate the production of omega 6 fatty acid (e.g. arachidonic acid or AA). The breakdown of AA to its metabolites leads to cancer growth, inflammation, immune dysfunction, cardiac disease, and neurologic illnesses such as the dementias – essentially all the calamities that may befall mankind.

"Our animal-protein-oriented society not only contributes inappropriately to global warming, but it also is a major source of AA, as well as total body acidification. The latter leads to bone loss with an associated release of bone-derived growth factors, a release that favors the acceleration of malignant growth, and every other malady mentioned above.

"There has been little or no emphasis on changing the predominant way we eat to a plant-based diet. There has been essentially no utilization of alkalinization to alter bone physiology and improve bone density while decreasing bone loss and preventing calcification in blood vessels (coronary arteries, aorta); tissues (kidney, prostate); and bladder stones and gallstones. There is compelling literature that we can decrease the incidence of PC as well as presentations of *aggressive* PC through the proactive use of selenium, vitamin E forms such as d-alpha tocopherol succinate, and gamma tocopherol, lycopene and boron. Despite this, it is rare to see men newly diagnosed with PC who have used a comprehensive dietary and/or supplement approach to avoid the entire problem of PC. Either the patient community requires a lot more education or the healthcare profession and the associated media need to do a lot more public relations work on this matter."

Q. So first of all, are there things we should avoid in our food? Why are they bad news for PC?

A. As mentioned above, in his book, 'Eating Your Way to Better Health' (see Recommended Reading), Dr Charles Myers discusses in detail the subject of fat and PC. He refers to studies performed by the Harvard School of Public Health. They found that '. . . dietary fat did not influence the risk of localised PC, but did increase the risk of metastatic PC. When they examined specific foods, red meat, dairy fat, egg yolk and creamy salad dressings emerged as significant risk factors for metastatic disease.'

Cancer progression can be spurred by eating red meat and milk products, according to a report in Medical News Today, 14 November 2008. In particular, meat heated to high temperatures – such as is usually done at a BBQ – contains heterocyclic amines or HCAs (Shirai et al., 2000) and charring of food such as charcoal-broiled or smoked foods, generates polycyclic aromatic hydrocarbons, or PAHs (Wilkinson G, 1997). These compounds are considered to be contra-indicated for PC patients – see Professor Avni Sali's comments below.

Sugar and other high Glycaemic Index foods are strongly contra-indicated in PC (Ewer, 2008). Products made with refined flours or refined grains, alcohol (except red wine, see in Ch 5), sweets, candies, cookies, cakes and pies should be consumed in limited amounts (Ledesma, 2005).

Professor Avni Sali, Director of the National Institute of Integrative Medicine in Australia, has provided a brief overview of the foodstuffs we should avoid in relation to

PC. In an article on the management of prostate cancer in Australian Doctor (September 4th, 2007), he wrote the following:

Fat

There is good evidence to associate prostate cancer with the Western diet, which is typically high in saturated animal fat and low in vegetables, fruit, fish and soy. Saturated fat, especially animal fat, is a risk factor for prostate cancer.

Dairy products increase the risk of prostate cancer. Calcium can suppress vitamin D by reducing the production of parathyroid hormone, and may explain the increased prostate cancer risk with dairy product consumption.

There is some controversy about whether omega-6 fats, especially when hydrogenated, increase the risk of prostate cancer.

Essential fatty acids from fish inhibit the growth of prostate cancer cells both in vitro and in vivo. Several epidemiological studies support an inverse association between consumption of fatty acids from fish and prostate cancer.

A study of scientific literature on the role of the fatty acid alpha-linolenic acid (ALA) in prostate cancer showed the risk of developing the disease increased with a high intake or higher blood level of ALA. Paradoxically, flaxseeds, which contain ALA, significantly reduce tumour proliferation rates in prostate cancer patients.

Monounsaturated fats reduce the risk of death from prostate cancer.

Red meat

It is likely that red meat consumption is associated with an increased risk of developing prostate cancer. Well-done meat contains heterocyclic amine and has been associated with colorectal and breast cancer. There is controversy as to whether the heterocyclic amine content of cooked meat increases prostate cancer risk, although an increased risk has been observed with an increased consumption of well-done red meat. High-fat and high red-meat diets, which tend to be low in plant foods, are likely to increase cancer risk.

Q. Which foods or food components are really helpful in preventing or attacking prostate cancer?

A. The Prostate Cancer Lifestyle Trial was conducted in 2001 in the USA to investigate the effect of dietary and other changes on the progression of PC. The results indicated that after one year, patients in the 'treatment' group showed small but significant decrease in PSA levels compared with controls. A later study followed the same patients for a further year. The results reinforced the first outcome.

Building on this promising foundation in 2005 Dr Dean Ornish and colleagues at University of California San Francisco campus, recruited 93 patients with biopsy-proven PC (PSA 4 to 10ng/ml and Gleason score <7). Half the men entered into an intensive program of nutritional modification, exercise and stress reduction, while the control group continued under normal care.

PSA decreased by 4% in the treatment group but increased by 6% in the control group. Growth of PC cells treated with serum from the treatment group was inhibited about 8 times more than when treated with serum from the control group.

The regime undertaken by the treatment group consisted of a diet which was effectively 'vegan', supplemented with soy protein powder, fish oil, vitamin E, selenium and vitamin C, together with moderate exercise – 30 min walking six days a week – and yoga-based stretching, breathing and relaxation/meditation.

In 2005 also, Dr Gordon Saxe and others from the University of California San Diego campus (UCSF), recruited 14 patients with recurrent PC – that is, their PSA began to rise after surgery or radiation. Patients entered a program of plant-based diet and stress reduction. The 'pre-post design' meant that each patient served as his own control. That is to say, patients were monitored as to baseline PSA level before the experiment began, then at the end of the intervention which was six months. There was a significant decrease in the rate of PSA rise from pre-study levels to six month levels. Four of ten evaluable patients had an absolute reduction in the PSA levels. Nine of ten had a reduction in their rates of rise of PSA and an improvement in their PSA doubling times, which increased from a median 12 months pre-study to 112 months post-intervention.

The UCSF group mentioned above took a major step forward in 2008. With similar intensive life-style interventions, Professor Ornish and colleagues demonstrated that it was possible even to change the way that genes behave in men with low-risk PC. Their elegant use of 'significance analysis of micro-arrays' demonstrated that the intervention switched on tumour killers and turned down tumour promoters. These surprising diet-gene interactions went a long way to explaining the molecular mechanisms behind the now well-established impact of nutrition on cancer.

Co-author and geneticist, Dr Christopher Haqq stated at a Scientific American News Conference (reported by Dr C Paddock, Medical News Today, June 18th 2008), that 'it is remarkable that such a straightforward life-style change can have as much effect as the most powerful drugs available . . .' Professor Ornish expressed surprise at how little time the 'treatment' took to work. He said, 'These changes can occur so quickly you don't have to wait years to see the benefits.'

It should be noted that in all of these life-style approaches, real improvements were reported in general health and feelings of well-being as well as in cardiovascular parameters.

Abundant scientific literature supports the healthy nature of the following foods, both for cardiovascular health and for cancer patients. Some are specifically valuable for PC as will be noted.

Professor Sali (quoted above) makes the following suggestions:

Vegetables and fruit

Vegetable consumption is likely to protect against prostate cancer. In the Physicians' Health Study, high plasma levels of lycopene, resulting primarily from a high intake of cooked tomatoes, were associated with a reduced risk of prostate cancer.

Recently, the US Food and Drug Administration stated that lycopene was not associated with a reduced risk of prostate, lung, colorectal, breast, cervical or endometrial cancer. Subsequently, Professor Giovannucci, professor of nutrition and epidemiology at HarvardUniversity, has defended the role of lycopene in the prevention of prostate cancer.

The consumption of legumes and yellow-orange and cruciferous vegetables is inversely related to the risk of developing prostate cancer. In general, multiple servings of fruit have also been shown to be inversely related to the progression of prostate cancer.

Pomegranate juice is a major source of phytochemicals. When consumed by men with a rising PSA after surgery or radiotherapy for prostate cancer, it was seen to cause a statistically significant prolonged PSA doubling time.

Soy

The major difference between Asian and US diets is the amount of soy-based foods consumed. The beneficial effects of soy have been attributed to isoflavones, in particular genistein and daidzein. In addition, soy phytoestrogens have a hormonal influence.

Soy isoflavones inhibit prostate cell growth in vitro, and in animal experiments. In a human study, phyto-oestrogens were shown to cause significant prostate cancer cell apoptosis (cell suicide).

Tea

Tea, especially green tea, is thought to inhibit cellular proliferation and induction of apoptosis and thus inhibit carcinogenesis or the development of cancer.

In a recent study, green tea polyphenols were shown to provide chemoprevention of prostate cancer in volunteers with high-grade prostate intraepithelial neoplasia. Green tea polyphenols selectively inhibit the COX-2 receptors in prostate cancer cells.

Fish

Fish is rich in protein and omega-3 fatty acids which are needed to restore the balance of omega-6 to omega-3. This balance is usually disturbed in western diets and PC patients in particular. Fish should be eaten often during the week and ideally replaces red meat.

Further nutritional information.

Cruciferous vegetables such as broccoli, Brussels sprouts, cabbage, bok choy. Chemical compounds called glucosinolates which occur in these vegetables, can inhibit, retard, or even reverse experimental multistage carcinogenesis (Fimognari 2002 LEF p42). When such foods are chewed (preferably uncooked or partly cooked), 'isothiocyanates' including sulforaphane are produced. Sulforaphane promotes apoptosis, induces specific enzymes in the liver which detoxify dangerous substances, and plays a role in the cell growth cycle (Ewer, 2008).

It is fortunate that 100grams of broccoli sprouts contain as much sulforaphane as a kilogram or more of the mature plant (Fahey et al., 1997). All of the above compounds from the Brassica vegetables have been shown to to have a role in the prevention and treatment of PC.

Multigrain breads Not only do these breads have a moderately low GI, but they usually contain seeds of various kinds such as sesame or linseed as well as plenty of fibre. Some contain additives such as soy and selenium. If toast is desired, it should not have any 'burn'.

Rolled oats or muesli as breakfast cereal. Low GI honey (such as Yellow Box or Manuka in Australia) as sweetener if necessary.

Cows' milk Given the dangers associated with this product for PC sufferers (Allen et al., 2008; Myers, 2000 p13), soy milk has great therapeutic advantages (Wahlquist, 2004).

Spreads such as olive oil (or spreads with no trans-fatty acids) may be used sparingly rather than butter or margarine.

Green tea (see under Supplements)

Snacks If these are desired, low GI biscuits or other similar are best. My wife makes a very healthy chocolate cake and very healthy biscuits.

Drinks/beverages Soy milks, cocoa, red wine in moderation, vegetable juice.

In Dr Charles Myers' book, 'Eating Your Way to Better Health' (see Recommended Reading) which is an excellent guide to diet/nutrition for PC patients, Myers sets out the biochemical rationale for his approach, including a valuable section on the 'Mediterranean diet'. The second part of the book by his wife, consists of recipes for tasty, prostate-healthy meals and snacks.

It might be helpful to mention just a few of the dishes which my own wife prepares: Lentil/pea/tomato soup, stir fry including tuna, sardines (in tomato sauce) on toast, brown or Basmati rice, chappatis made from wholemeal flour, falafels (made from chick peas). Egg white is fine and where eggs are required in a recipe, 'Egg replacer' is useful. If sweeteners are desired, stevia is acceptable, low GI honey etc., Nicola and sweet potatoes have a low GI. We have fish often, chicken once a week or so, red meat more rarely and then not over-done.

Among our desserts there would be very healthy chocolate bread pudding, soy yoghurt, fresh fruit salad (not commercial tinned fruit in syrup etc.), Basmati rice and prunes. Many of our preparations are either from Myers' book or are adaptations of them.

Other foods/nutrients which should ideally be incorporated into our menu include: capsicum (red chilli peppers), turmeric (curcumin), garlic and cloves, brown or Basmati rice, whole grains and legumes such as peas, beans and nuts, tomato products such as tomato sauce and paste, fruits, particularly apples which contain pectin.

In Chapter 5 on supplements, we will consider further phytonutrients. Some of these are discussed in Appendix 3 for the advanced reader.

Q. If diet is a big issue, I'm afraid my husband will not be happy! He loves his bacon and eggs, pavlova, cream and all that. I will need help!

A. (By my wife Elizabeth.) Well, my husband used to love bacon and eggs, steak, roast lamb and so on. His new-found interest in his health, however, changed all that. Now he has a largely vegetarian diet and enjoys it greatly.

He has more energy and is far healthier in all ways. He has cut out nearly all the medications he used to take, such as statins for cholesterol, sulfasalazine and paracetamol for arthritic pain, betamethasone for psoriasis. Salt has been virtually eliminated, though we do use a little 'low salt' which is potassium chloride instead of sodium chloride. He still has high blood pressure but takes fewer tablets than before.

He also has a sweet tooth although he has trained himself to accept and enjoy less sweetening. Where they are really needed, we use the appropriate substitutes.

Q. A friend told me about caloric restriction'. What is that about?

A. This was mentioned above (Dr Strum). There is a growing literature supporting the notion that not only is obesity a very bad thing for PC, keeping the calories down is extremely helpful. It is thought that a caloric intake of less than 2000/day is the aim; that is, about 8,400 Joules. It must be emphasised, however, that common sense must prevail, because a sick survivor is no use to himself or others. One's medical advisors and support person or friends will be helpful here.

Q. What is 'juicing'?

A. Freshly made concentrated vegetable juice is full of polyphenols and other anti-oxidants as well as chlorophyll/ chlorophyllin together with valuable enzymes, vitamins, minerals and many other nutrients. We get fibre from other sources.

We use a hand juicer rather than a vitamizer or blender, since these can generate much heat which destroys many of the enzymes and other nutrients in the juice. Commercial vegetable juices are often useful.

Q. I'm a bit overweight. Does that matter?

A. Yes it does. Particularly for PC sufferers.

Professor Sali, in the article for Australian Doctor mentioned above, wrote the following:

'The evidence regarding obesity increasing the risk of prostate cancer is still unclear but tends to support a link. A recent study showed that a high BMI – that is, Body Mass Index – with weight gain is associated with a greater risk of mortality from prostate cancer.

It is of interest that Asian men in the US have a better prostate cancer survival rate, which could be due to their lower weight.'

Ideally the man's BMI should be in the low twenties, and waist or girth measurement should be less than 94cm.

Q. What is GL?

A. GI was mentioned above as a measure of how fast food is digested and therefore how much and how rapidly the blood sugar rises. The insulin surge which follows is bad for PC because insulin is a growth factor for PC cells.

Glycaemic Load is a measure of how much a particular serving of food will raise blood sugar. So while the GI might be high, if you have only a small amount it won't have much effect on blood sugar and therefore on insulin release. Conversely if you have a larger amount of a food with low GI it won't have much effect either.

Now in fact you don't need to weigh out the amount of food, calculate the available carbohydrate and so on. Generally speaking, if you wish to have a food with high GI, then don't have much of it, and combine with it a food which has a low GI. This more or less 'evens out' the overall GI. There are tables of foods and their GI and GL on the internet for those who wish to go deeper.

Q. I love my bacon and eggs. Is that OK? Occasionally?

A. What one eats once in a while is probably not going to be harmful. If a 'bad' food is eaten regularly, however, then the result will be bad. It is hard to define what 'once in a while' means exactly, but one rule of thumb is that at least 85% of our intake should be from the 'good end' of the spectrum.

Q. What is 'nutrigenomics'?

A. The new science of 'nutrigenomics' is the formal study of the way nutrition impacts on one's genes, or more precisely, on gene products. Molecular biology is a complex science which investigates all that's happening inside the cell. The present book is quite rudimentary, but the reader may be so enthralled that he or she decides to pursue the subject more fully and Appendix 3 and Recommended Reading are intended for that.

SUMMARY

The Take-Home Message is, take Hippocrates' advice and let food be your medicine.

Exercise self control at the table. Plan your menu according to well established models. Remember that 'Heart-healthy' is also 'Prostate-healthy'. Remember that caloric restriction is the way to health and longevity, but don't over-do it. Prepare your own meals if you can. Meals and their preparation should not only be healthy, but should be fun!

5

Supplements

'We now have a body of solid evidence,' writes Dr J Pinsky (2007), 'upon which to stand when we claim that natural ingredients can prolong prostate vitality . . . and prevent PC cells from developing . . . Natural dietary supplements are now part of standard treatment and prevention of prostate cancer.' He then proceeds to discuss the results of several studies conducted over the last decade at highly respected medical research institutions in the US and Europe, attesting to the efficacy of supplements in preventing PC and affecting PC cell growth.

From a nutritional point of view, we cancer patients may not be able to eat enough broccoli or whatever to achieve the optimum blood level of the active ingredients. In the case of broccoli, you would have to eat 200 grams or more a day to get the recommended amount of the compounds sulforaphane and carbinols. This is where supplements may be necessary – or in the case of broccoli, sprouts!

Different supplements have various levels of experimental underpinning for their reputations. Some are purely observational or 'epidemiological' and we don't really know how they work. Others, however, have strong scientific support and we do know the biochemical actions and specifically how they impact on cancer cells.

At the 2007 Prostate Cancer Symposium held in Toronto, Dr Neil Fleshner presented some fascinating data that build on previous studies showing anti-cancer benefits in men receiving selenium, lycopene or vitamin E. Dr Fleshner looked at the combination of all three agents administered to men who were scheduled to undergo radical prostatectomy. When all three agents were administered, uniformly favourable pathologic changes indicating slower growth and reduced metastatic potential were seen. These changes occurred within a matter of weeks of starting these common supplements. When men were treated with only one or two of these agents, the results were not nearly as good.

Kobyashi and colleagues in 2006 studied dietary fatty acid ratios in immunodeficient mice. These mice were injected with PC cells and then fed diets differing in the amounts of various fatty acids. Tumor growth, volume and PSA levels were later measured. The mice fed a diet richer in omega-3 fatty acids fared better than those fed with more omega-6 fatty acids. These results provide a sound basis for clinical trials evaluating the effect of dietary omega-3 fatty acids from fish oil on tumor PGE_2 and membrane fatty acid composition, and serum and tumor biomarkers of progression in men with prostate cancer.

It will now be a useful exercise to examine a few of the most important supplements in some detail. Their specific biological actions on PC – and other cancers too – will be briefly explained, with more technical detail in Appendix 3. The biochemical and molecular pathways which will be described are common to very many of the considerable range of phytonutrients or supplements. This is why a naturopath or clinician skilled in phytochemistry is advisable as a member of the PC medical team.

Vitamin D The scientific literature on Vitamin D and cancer is considerable and increasing rapidly. This vitamin – or more correctly, this 'hormone' – is so important in prostate cancer that the pathophysiology will be discussed before the Questions and Answers.

It is estimated that 50,000–63,000 individuals in the USA and 19,000–25,000 in the UK die prematurely from cancer annually due to insufficient vitamin D (Photochemistry Photobiology, 2005;81: 1276–1286.)

Recently it was reported that 1000–2000 IU of vitamin D obtained from sunlight exposure, dietary supplements or the diet, would cut the risk of colon cancer in half (Amer J Prevent Med. 2007;32: 210–216.)

A research team from the UCSD reported that vitamin D supplementation would reduce the occurrence of a wide variety of cancers by 30–50% (Amer J Pub Health, 2006;96: 252–261.)

Sunlight is the natural 'source' of Vitamin D. Various biochemical reactions occur first in the exposed skin, then in the liver, and then in the kidneys to produce 1,25-OH_2 vitamin D (or calcitriol). This is the most active form of the vitamin. In fact, according to oncologist Dr Charles Myers who has been mentioned above, the level of calcitriol is far more important than the level of calcidiol which is the one normally measured in a laboratory (Myers, 2007 p158).

It was reported recently that calcitriol, the active form of vitamin D, has been found to induce a tumor suppressing protein that can inhibit the growth of breast cancer cells (*Science Daily*, February 5th, 2009).

In line with this thinking, it has been suggested (Schwartz, 2008) that whereas the vitamin D form commonly used as a supplement might prevent PC, *existing* prostate tumours would probably need treatment with calcitriol. The reason for this is that many PC cells have lost the ability to synthesize calcitriol but still possess receptors for the hormone.

Because of the risk of skin cancer, sun exposure should be restricted to the hours before mid-morning and after mid-afternoon. Even then, exposure should not produce more than a faint reddening of the skin. The actual practise of sun exposure should be discussed with one's GP. Vitamin D is also available in capsules or tablet form, and dosage should also be with medical advice if this approach is chosen. A combination of sun-exposure and Vitamin D supplement is convenient but needs monitoring by pathology testing. You can't get too much Vitamin D from sunlight, but you *can* get toxicity from the supplements.

Thorough reviews about these properties and actions of vitamin D are available in several reports (Krishnan et al., 2003; Lamprecht et al., 2003; Hollick M, 2007; Ingraham et al., 2008; Grant M, 2009.) For more technical information see Appendix 3.

Q. I read that pomegranate juice is good for PC. Is this true, and if so how does it help?

A. A flurry of recent research activity has occurred on the action of this supplement in PC. Most men with the condition have heard of the remarkable results obtained by UCLA Department of Urology researchers. The recent history is as follows:

In 2004, Albrecht et al., showed that pomegranate extract potently suppressed growth, proliferation and invasion of human PC cells transplanted into an animal.

In 2005, Malik et al., extended the above work to study the molecular mechanisms by which these effects were produced.

In 2006, Dr A. Pantuck's team from UCLA monitored 50 PC patients who had undergone surgery or radiotherapy. These men still had cancer because their PSA had increased even after therapy. They were given pomegranate juice and the rate at which their PSA rose, decreased by 35% on average. The PSA doubling time increased in 80% of the men from 15 months to 54 months. When serum from these men was applied to PC cells in cultures, cell growth rate markedly decreased and cell death rate increased considerably.

It was found recently that pomegranate polyphenols down-regulate the expression of androgen-synthesizing genes in human prostate cancer cells which overexpress the androgen receptor (Young Hong et al., 2008). What this means is, that the ability of pomegranate to protect against cancer – and by extension, to aid in its treatment – may be due to direct interaction with genes.

Pantuck and colleagues recently did a follow-up of some of the participants in their original pomegranate study. During the six-year follow-up, men who continued drinking pomegranate juice had lower PSA levels than those who stopped drinking the juice and were no longer active in the trial. By the end of the study, it took about four times longer for active participants' PSA levels to double than it had at the beginning of the study (Pantuck et al., 2009).

Q. What about soy?

A. Isoflavones are polyphenols found in soy, lentils, peas, beans red clover and so on. Isoflavone consumption is associated with a low incidence of metastatic PC (Gaynor, 2003). The main components in isoflavones are genistein and daidzein, but there is more research evidence supporting the effect of genistein in PC.

Genistein is a phytoestrogen. The oestrogenic effects, however, are very mild compared with oestradiol, the main form of the hormone. The phytoestrogen occupies binding sites on the cells thus competing with oestradiol and rendering it less effective. There is considerable recent literature indicating that the actions of oestradiol contribute substantially to the development of PC (for example Giton et al., 2008; Singh et al., 2008). For the keener reader, Appendix 3 illustrates some of the ways in which genistein works.

Daidzein also has powerful actions but depends on its conversion to equol, and not everyone's metabolism can effect this.

Q. What other supplements are important in PC?

A. The following supplements are more or less representative of a vast array of useful herbs and other compounds. The few chosen are illustrative only and are not necessarily considered in order of their importance:

Green tea The common green tea is valuable, but to get the best results it is necessary to drink up to ten cups a day. It is more convenient to buy tablets or capsules containing little caffeine. The active ingredient, epigallocatechin gallate (EGCG) is anti-inflammatory and is a powerful anti-oxidant. It has many biochemical actions and the main effects from the point of view of PC are explained in Appendix 3.

Curcumin is a spice with a long history in the field of natural health compounds and a vast scientific literature underpinning its claimed actions. Epidemiological studies suggest that people who eat curcumin as a spice, have a lower incidence of cancer than others (Thangapazham et al. 2006). Both *in vivo* and *in vitro* experiments have demonstrated that curcumin (diferuloylmethane) can affect signalling steps critical for tumour growth and that it can inhibit initiation, promotion and invasion of tumours as well as angiogenesis and metastasis.

Silymarin is a chemical derived from St Mary's milk thistle and it has numerous actions against PC cells. Further information is to be found in Appendix 3.

Cinnamon is an interesting spice which deserves comment. It has been mentioned above that insulin spikes are a problem in PC. It has been found that taking half a teaspoon of cinnamon twice a day in whatever medium, effectively slows down absorption in the stomach and also improves insulin function and insulin resistance.

Cinnamon increases the amount of three critically important proteins involved in the body's insulin signalling, glucose transport and inflammatory response thus effectively potentiating insulin's action.

These data were presented at Experimental Biology as part of the American Society for Nutrition, Inc scientific program held in San Francisco, April 4th 2006.

Cocoa is a very rich source of antioxidants. Dark chocolate containing more than 70% cocoa is therefore a valuable supplement but only in sensible amounts – up to 50 grams per day. Cocoa generates endorphins, the body's natural mood enhancers, and it contains relaxing compounds which may reduce stress.

Due to the extraordinary amount of phenolic phytochemicals it contains, cocoa kills cancer cells and protects against heart disease. It also contains high levels of chromium, zinc and magnesium and this may explain a normalising effect on blood sugar.

Pomegranate see above and especially Appendix 3.

Quercetin is a bioflavanoid found in onions, nuts, berries, vegetables such as cabbage, fruit such as apples, grains and wine. It is a well-known anti-oxidant, and of recent times its potential anti-cancer activity has brought it into prominence.

Resveratrol Found in red wine, peanuts, some berries. See Appendix 3 for further information.

Selenium It is thought perhaps not as effective in preventing the initiation of PC but is highly effective in slowing down tumour progression (Li et al., 2004; Taylor et al., 2004). Dr Graham Lyons from the University of Adelaide has written an informative article on the role of selenium and other nutrients in PC (Lyons, 2009).

He makes the point that in the case of green tea, tomato and pomegranate, studies have generally found that the food/whole forms (supplied in suitable amounts) were more effective against prostate cancer than purified extracts of the (supposedly) main active agents.

Selenium as selenite has recently been shown to have great therapeutic potential against multi-drug resistant cancer cells (Olm et al., 2009).

See also Appendix 3.

Serenoa (Saw palmetto) See Appendix 3 for further information.

Vitamin C There has been conflicting evidence as to the efficacy of Vitamin C in PC, but recent evidence demonstrates its synergistic action with vitamin K3 (Tareen et al., 2008). This group treated seventeen patients – who had failed standard therapy – with 5000mg vitamin C and 50mg vitamin K3 daily, for 12 weeks. At the conclusion of the 12 week treatment period, PSA velocity decreased and PSA doubling time increased in 13 of 17 patients ($p \leq 0.05$). There were no dose-limiting adverse effects. For further clarification of terms, see Appendix 3.

Of the 15 patients who continued on therapy after 12 weeks, only 1 death occurred after 14 months of treatment, and these were patients with aggressive cancer. Treatment dose was doubled for the three participants who showed no initial response, and this achieved the desired result.

Vitamin E (as natural tocopherols and tocotrienols) There

are eight isoforms of Vitamin E, four tocopherols and four tocotrienols, and growing evidence suggests that the latter may be more important in cancer than the former. The so-called 'natural' Vitamin E (d-alpha tocopherol) commonly sold may not be the best form to take for addressing PC. In fact the isoform gamma-tocopherol is much more efficacious. Gamma-tocopherol has also been shown to boost the protective effects of both alpha-tocopherol and selenium. Compared with individuals with low concentrations of all three micronutrients, high concentrations of selenium and alpha-tocopherol were associated with a statistically significant decreased risk of prostate cancer only when high concentrations of gamma-tocopherol were also present (Daily University Science News, 21st December, 2001).

Wright et al., (2007) showed that supplemental vitamin E intake was not related to prostate cancer risk overall. However, dietary γ-tocopherol was significantly inversely related to advanced disease. This inverse association was particularly evident among men with low selenium intake. They also demonstrated that the gamma form was associated with a significant reduction in the risk of advanced prostate cancer.

Recent research suggested that γ-tocotrienol was most potent in suppressing prostate cancer cell proliferation, and that the antiproliferative effect of γ-tocotrienol acts through multiple-signalling pathways. In addition, the same study demonstrated the anti-invasion and chemosensitisation effect of γ-tocotrienol against PC cells (Yap et al., 2008). For a brief discussion on the cancellation of a recent vitamin E trial, see Appendix 3.

Coenzyme Q10 This is a vitamin-like nutrient found in all cells of the body, in the 'power house' or mitochrondia. It is a powerful antioxidant, it boosts energy and enhances the immune system.

In terms of its action on cancer, CoQ10 as it is known, significantly reduces bcl-2 which effectively encourages apoptosis. The body's level of CoQ10 can be depleted as by aging, cancer, or by statins, medications used to lower cholesterol. Maintaining adequate intake – perhaps with supplements – is therefore advisable for those with cancer.

A Danish team of cancer specialists achieved remarkable results with breast cancer patients following the use of CoQ10 therapy. They treated 32 high risk breast cancer patients with antioxidants including daily CoQ10. The disease progression rate was surprisingly modified, and it soon became clear that is was the coenzyme which was the main driver (Lockwood et al., 1994). One year later, follow-up study confirmed the on-going results and revealed that some subjects had complete remission with tumours disappearing and no evidence of metastases (Lockwood et al., 1995).

Fish oil (take only products which are free of mercury, and ideally free of aldehydes and lipid peroxides) Contains EPA and DHA, important omega-3 fatty acids. These modulate eicosanoid synthesis (see above), and they influence gene expression, receptor function and cell-signalling all of which play a critical role in the progression of PC.

It has recently been shown that the omega fatty acid balance can alter immunity and gene expression, both of which of course have tremendous significance in PC. This was reported in Medical News Today, 4th June, 2009.

An excellent overview of natural health products (NHPs) is provided by Yance and Sagar (2006). The authors focus on NHPs that have a high degree of antiangiogenic activity but also describe some of their many other interactions that can inhibit tumor progression and reduce the risk of metastases. See Appendix 3 for more.

Q. Buying and taking all these supplements looks really complicated, doesn't it?

A. At first glance it would seem so. However, many patients will appreciate knowing that there is a capsule commercially available which includes the main chemical compounds such as herbs. It is called Prostasol. Two versions are available, one from the UK and another from Seacoast Vitamins in the USA. It should be said that Prostasol, while available without prescription from the UK and America, should not be taken without medical supervision.

Prostasol has a very interesting history. A herbal product called PC-SPES was available until 2002 and it produced quite remarkable reduction of PSA levels in patients. Urologists around the world were adopting it. Unfortunately, it was found to contain traces of diethylstilbestrol which can cause blood clots, and the FDA recommended that it be withdrawn from sale. The compound also had traces of warfarin and indomethacin.

For some years this situation continued, until the two versions of Prostasol appeared. The benefits of PC-SPES were maintained in both without the contaminants and the associated risks, and each contained two additional compounds. Because the herbs in Prostasol have such a remarkable effect, and because their mode of action nicely illustrates the power of 'alternative' or 'complementary' medicines in PC, it is worth looking at the components in some detail. It should not be a surprise that the effect of all the ingredients combined together, has been shown to be superior to that of individual compounds.

Constituents of Prostasol (Seacoast USA variety, also called QuercetinPlus):

Serenoa repens (saw palmetto) This compound is commonly taken by men with BPH (Benign Prostatic Hyperplasia) or enlargement of the prostate. It is a 'phytoestrogen', or oestrogen mimic which can bind competitively to oestrogen receptors without producing the strong negative effects of oestradiol.

Sterolin mix Sterols are plant compounds with strong immunomodulatory effects. The sterols need to act with their glycosides – sterolins – for best effect. These phytosterols are known to inhibit 5-alpha reductase and also aromatase which converts testosterone to estrogen.

Beta-sitosterol inhibits the growth of human PC cells.

Quercetin is a flavonoid with powerful effects against 'reactive oxygen species', modulates gene expression and acts as a calmodulin antagonist. Calmodulin is a calcium binding agent which plays an important role in prostate cancer progression.

Boron as boric acid decreased PSA levels by 87% and reduced tumor size in a prostate cancer mouse model. Mice receiving 1.7 or 9.0 mg/kg/day of boric acid solution orally had decreases in tumor size by 38% and 25%, respectively.

The same groups had drops in PSA of 88.6% and 86.4%, respectively. The control group receiving only water had no drop in PSA or decrease in tumor size. This was reported in Proc. Amer. Assoc. Cancer Res. 2002;43:77.

Nattokinase is an enzyme extracted from natto, which itself is a form of fermented soy. Nattokinase contains vitamin K2 (a menaquinone) which is known to inhibit cancer cell growth for liver, lung, stomach and breast tumors. A recent study clarified the link between the dietary intake of vitamin K and prostate cancer protection (Nimptsch, K. et al. *Am. J. Clin. Nutr.* 2008;87:985-92.)

Japanese scientists recently showed that natto (and viscous vegetables) were found to suppress postprandial glucose and insulin responses (Yamanaka et al., 2008).

Reishi is a potent mushroom (ganoderma lucidum). See Appendix 3 for further information.

Pygeum has been shown to have anti-mitogenic action. That is to say, it tends to stop the cancer cells from dividing. See Appendix 3.

Ginger, or more exactly 6-gingerol, induces cell cycle arrest via multiple mechanisms. It has particularly strong anti-5-LOX action and it is a powerful 'apoptotic' (Seong-Ho L et al., 2007). These authors offer an hypothesis based on their experiments, as to the mechanisms of action of gingerol, see Appendix 3.

Panax ginseng has various functions including mitotic activity towards T cells – that is, it stimulates the immune system. It also has anti-carcinogenic effects. See Appendix 3.

Curcumin has numerous effects on cellular events which impact strongly on PC. The effects have been documented in a prolific literature and include inhibition of cell proliferation, induction of apoptosis, and inhibition of angiogenesis of LNCaP prostate cancer cells in vivo. See Appendix 3.

Prostasol can be taken in conjunction with other primary therapies, but of course it is essential to discuss the matter with one's (integrative) medical advisors. It is, as always, essential to maintain a healthy diet and lifestyle and if required, to take other supplements as well such as green tea, selenium and the other compounds mentioned above.

Q. How can we know that the PSA lowering effect is not an artifact? That is, could the herbs be affecting just the biomarker and not the cancer?

A. Firstly, by-and-large the cellular errors and molecular events which happen in the initiation and progression of PC are known and pretty well understood. These, the reader may remember, involve *hormonal balance*, *cell signalling*, *cell cycle regulation*, *cell survival*, *cellular differentiation*, *angiogenesis*, and *metabolism of potential carcinogens* as discussed in Chapter 4.

We also now understand the biochemical mechanisms by which most of the compounds mentioned in this book operate. It was mentioned above that Professor Dean Ornish has demonstrated that diet and lifestyle can even change the way our genes express their products. The diet had added supplements such as soy, fish oil, vitamin E, selenium and vitamin C. Concentrated herbal activity such as is found in Prostasol – together with the other Ornish lifestyle elements – can be expected to be at least as powerful.

For example, consider again the enzyme 5-Lipoxygenase (5-LOX) which was mentioned above. 5-LOX converts the fatty acid arachidonic acid which is found in our diet, into a compound called 5-HETE. Prostate cancer cells need 5-HETE to survive, so inhibiting this compound will negatively impact prostate cancer.

Prostasol contains four ingredients – serenoa, quercetin, gingerol and curcumin – which are known to have strong action against this critical enzyme.

Prostasol has only minimal side effects, notably some diminishing of libido and slight gynecomastia or slightly enlarged breasts with mild nipple tenderness. Now these symptoms occur, though more markedly, together with significant other problems when men have 'Androgen Blockade' or 'Androgen Deprivation' therapy. This hormonal therapy is normally reserved for men with advanced PC who have failed primary interventions.

The significance of this similarity, is that the effects which occur in common are due to blocking of the androgen receptor (AR). Therefore in this respect, Prostasol is somewhat like hormonal therapy without the very unpleasant accompaniments to the conventional medications. In fact the mild adverse effects on the breasts and nipples in men may be due either to the activity of unopposed oestrogen, or to deficiency of oestrogen, but we will not go further into the discussion here.

The AR plays quite a critical part in PC. Normally the AR has to be complexed with an androgen to stimulate PC cells. However, the receptor has various way of adapting to the absence of testosterone or dihydrotestosterone, DHT. As indicated above, metastatic prostate cancer is treated with drugs that antagonize the action of androgens, but most patients progress to a more aggressive form of the disease called androgen independent prostate cancer which is driven by elevated expression of the androgen receptor. That is why other drugs are sought which will negatively impact the AR. Prostasol does this.

Secondly, when PC-SPES appeared, a plethora of papers came out between the years 1995 and 2002, documenting the remarkable benefits of the herbal mix. These were not just lowering of PSA, but real clinical effects such as reduction of bone pain in men with metastases. Unfortunately, when the product had to be recalled, the articles dried up very quickly. Only a few researchers kept up the studies, first on PC-SPES and then some of these laboratories and clinics decided to generate a modified product with basically the same herbs, but without the contaminants. So Prostasol was born.

Cancer Research UK in its 2007 'CancerHelp' review of PC-SPES and a similar product called PC-HOPE, advised that the compounds be kept as a 'fall-back' in case conventional hormonal therapy fails. These compounds contained the same compounds as Prostasol and it is stated that PC-SPES could:

- Lower PSA and testosterone levels
- Reduce bone pain in one third of men with this symptom
- Shrink prostate tumors significantly in some men.

The American Cancer Society (ACS) has also written an overview of PC-SPES and similar compounds (including Prostasol). It states the following about the products in its web-site 'Making Treatment Decisions, 2007':

> *Several carefully designed clinical trials found that PC-SPES was an effective treatment for patients with PC, including some whose cancer did not respond to conventional hormone therapy . . .*
>
> *PC-SPES has been carefully evaluated in several clinical trials. In virtually all of these studies PC-SPES was found to be effective in reducing blood levels of PSA. Some studies have also observed tumors to shrink following treatment.*
>
> *A randomised trial comparing PC-SPES with DES (diethylstilboestrol) was started before problems with contamination were known, and results were published in 2004. DES is sometimes used as a hormonal treatment for PC that is no longer responding to hormone therapy . . . the herbal product was actually more effective than DES in lowering PSA and in delaying growth of the cancer. The men taking PC-SPES were less likely than those taking DES to develop blood clots.*

A comprehensive article on the effectiveness of PC-SPES is that by Ades et al., (2001). These authors thoroughly review the clinical data and offer a good reference list for those interested in understanding the interest generated by the product in the medical – especially the urological – community.

Darzynkiewicz (2000) examined the mechanisms behind the obvious clinical effectiveness of PC-SPES.

He concluded that this was likely due to its complex composition, which probably targeted many signal transduction and metabolic pathways simultaneously, thereby eliminating the back-up or redundant mechanisms that otherwise promote cell survival when single-target agents are used.

Thirdly, Professor Ben Pfeifer, the Swiss oncologist who pioneered the development of Prostasol, conducted thorough basic and clinical trials with surprising results. It is well worth studying one of these briefly, not to promote the compound, but to illustrate the effectiveness of these herbs and other phytochemicals of a similar nature and to address the 'artifact' question.

In one study, Pfeifer and colleagues treated men with advanced hormone refractory PC. Within a few months of taking 900 to 2800mg of Prostasol, a drop of more than 50% in the PSA reading occurred in approximately 70% of the men. The results were not published in a peer-reviewed journal, but can be found through a Google search using Professor Ben Pfeifer and Prostasol as key words. Pfeifer and colleagues at the Aesculap Klinik in Switzerland report that this sort of decrease is often associated with a decline in metastatic pain and a general improvement in quality of life. In about one third of these hormone refractory patients, there was a decrease in tumour mass in the primary tumour and/or the metastases.

Although Prostasol is the mainstay of the Pfeifer regime, immune therapy is also used as well as treatment with curcumin and a combination of other herbs such as green tea extract.

Fourthly, there is considerable scientific argument that the PSA itself is not simply a biomarker, and that it is produced by the PC cells to 'further their own cause' (Falloon and Strum, 2005–2006). The antigen breaks down proteins (Webber et al., 1995) and, it is thought, this may be a mechanism to enable invasion into the extracellular matrix or complex biological glue which holds cells in place. It was found recently (Yuanjie et al., 2008) that tissue PSA seems to facilitate very aggressive prostate tumour progression by its action on the AR and subsequent down-modulating of the cancer suppressor, p53.

Given this strong evidence, it would therefore seem medically responsible to reduce PSA levels as the above authors suggest.

It has also been noticed of recent years that aspirin and statins – medication commonly prescribed for the control of cholesterol – can lower the PSA level in men. This has raised the question we are now addressing – could it be that the medications are acting at a level which reduces the production of the PSA but without acting on the development or progression of the tumour? In other words, could they be masking an undetected cancer or progression of an existing one, thus putting lives at risk?

I am not aware of any evidence to date that this has ever happened, but in this new ultra hi-tech era perhaps trials could be designed to resolve the matter. It would be necessary to recruit men with diagnosed PC who have not had treatment or who are not responding to treatment.

Baselines would need to be established, treatment protocols carefully designed and monitored. The men would begin taking Abiraterone, a statin or Prostasol or other compound known to suppress PSA. Then repeat biopsies or monitoring of other markers or procedures might be performed to study histopathological changes or more sophisticated gene expression as done by Ornish et al., 2008. PSA changes such as PSADT would be followed, since this parameter is considered to be the single most reliable indicator of PC progression (McLaren et al., 1998). Each participant would be acting as his own control, pre-intervention/post-intervention. See further Appendix 3.

Nogueira et al., (2009) have reviewed the various biomarkers which could be used to monitor for advancing PC including recent novel assays.

From all of the above, it would seem unlikely that masking is happening, but it would be a nice experiment and it might put doubts to rest.

Other supplements still need to be taken separately, but at least the Prostasol capsule reduces the number of tablets/drops/powders to be taken. Also it is highly doubtful that any 'home-made' mix will be as good as this commercial preparation.

For more in-depth, technical discussion of the Ornish results and their significance to this question, as well as for further evidence see Appendix 3.

Nutritional supplements (Sali)

Selenium

Epidemiological studies have found that low levels of plasma selenium are associated with an increased incidence of prostate cancer.

In a 10-year double-blind study, selenium taken as a supplement (200ug) reduced the incidence of prostate cancer by 52%, and it was especially protective in those with the lowest serum selenium levels.

Vitamin E

Vitamin E, even in small doses, offers protection against prostate cancer.

In the Alpha-Tocopherol, Beta-Carotene Cancer Prevention Study of 29,133 men, there was a 32% reduction in the incidence of prostate cancer among those males who received vitamin E (alpha-tocopherol 50mg). Vitamin E inhibits human prostate cancer cell growth by modulating the cell cycle regulatory machinery.

The gamma forms of tocopherol and tocotrienol are the most effective.

Vitamin D

Numerous studies have reported an inverse association between ultraviolet light exposure and mortality rates for prostate cancer.

Analysis of the serum from 250,000 subjects found that low vitamin D was a risk factor for prostate cancer.

Receptors for vitamin D exist on human prostate cancer cells. Prostate cancer patients who have the highest levels of vitamin D have a better prognosis.

Curcumin

Curcumin is known to be a COX-2 inhibitor and can induce apoptosis of prostate cancer cells, as well as enhancing cytotoxicity of chemotherapeutic agents, and conferring a radiosensitising effect on prostate cancer cells.

Herbal supplements

A Chinese herbal combination called PC-SPES that contains eight herbs has been found to influence prostate cancer and reduce PSA levels. But this US product was found to be contaminated and was banned.

A similar product, Prostasol, which contains no contaminants, is currently available overseas. Very little is known about interactions between Prostasol and conventional medications. Caution is prudent when using any supplements with pharmaceutical products.

SUMMARY

The Take-Home Message is, get what your body needs from simple, healthy food. Ask your advisors as to what supplements you need beyond that.

If I had to give you my personal choice for the main supplements which cannot be done without, it would be Vitamin D – from the sun for preference – followed closely by fish oil. Your holistic medical team will advise you further.

6

Exercise

The benefits of exercise are well known. Exercise influences our cardiovascular system, keeps weight down, improves our mental and emotional state. In terms of cancer, however, the effects are quite fundamental and we now know many of the mechanisms involved.

In a recent study, men 65 and older who exercised regularly for about 3 hours a week reduced their risk of advanced PC by nearly 70% (reported in The Johns Hopkins on-line Health Report, 11th February 2009). About 30 minutes of moderate exercise a day is desirable, though if the activity is more intense, less time would be acceptable. The very process of doing something enjoyable which requires effort, effectively 'takes you away' at least for a short time into a healthier dimension of being (Sali, 2006).

As indicated earlier, the diagnosis of prostate (or any other) cancer is almost always a cause of depression. Men may not complain to their doctor about it, and may not even be aware that they are suffering from depression. They put up with the sleeplessness or the 'feeling blue', the lack of appetite and so on and may consider it just part of the condition. Certainly none of my medical advisors – apart from my current urologist and the Integrative Medicine specialist – raised the matter with me.

The depression is harmful to the psyche of the individual of course, but it will also impact on one's immune system. Ohio State University researchers found an exaggerated inflammatory response among people feeling stressed and suffering 'subclinical' depression. Following a single flu shot, their bodies overproduced the immune system component interleukin-6, a marker of long-term inflammation and well known to be bad news for prostate cancer sufferers. This was reported in the November 1st, 2003 *Newsletter of Psychology Today*, 'Depression Hurts the Immune System'.

Should a doctor realise that his/her prostate cancer patient is suffering from depression, the high probability is that anti-depressant medication will be prescribed. That is not to say that this is an incorrect way to go. However, this approach will generally take a few weeks to establish the most appropriate drug. Then, as if the patient doesn't already have enough problems, there is a latent period before the therapeutic dose level is achieved and there are usually attendant side effects, sometimes quite unpleasant.

So while it is not the intention here to down-play the value of pharmacology in such a setting, there are other ways. Such as exercise!

Stress and depression may impair a cancer patient's body's ability to fight off infection and potentially to deal with the progression of the disease, Stanford University School of Medicine's Dr David Spiegel wrote in an August 2009 Newsletter. Between 15 and 25 percent of cancer patients experience major depression, marked by feelings of hopelessness, helplessness, worthlessness, fatigue and loss of interest in daily life. Depression may make cancer patients' prognosis worse: studies have shown that higher levels of depression correlate with faster tumor growth.

"What investigators at Stanford have done is begin to identify the mechanisms for the relationship between depression and a worse outcome in cancer," said Emory University School of Medicine psychiatrist Andrew Miller, MD, who also directs a psychiatric oncology program in Atlanta.

It was reported in *Science Daily*, November 30th 1999, that depression alters the immune system by decreasing physical activity. Most of us have an intuitive appreciation of this, because anyone who has run for a reasonable distance notices a lifting of the spirit – indeed long distance runners experience such a 'feel-good' rush that it has been likened to euphoria. This is surely a clue as to the value of exercise.

Dr James Gordon, eminent psychiatrist and Director of the Center for Mind-Body Medicine in Washington DC, is an ardent promoter of exercise in the treatment of depression. In his book, *Unstuck: Your Guide to the Seven Stage Journey out of Depression* (Penguin Press, 2008), he explains in Chapter 3 with its associated Notes, that exercise actually alters brain chemistry for the better. It causes an increase in serotonin as well as endorphin levels. It reduces neuroendocrine stress hormones and decreases peoples' depression scores.

Dr Gordon recommends a variety of exercises including dancing, but states that jogging has been most studied in terms of effectiveness compared with anti-depressant medications. He states that 'this sense of being active on our own behalf may be . . . the single, most direct and powerful antidote to the feeling of hopelessness and helplessness that are hallmarks of depression.' (p162)

Q. List some other ways in which exercise impacts on PC.

A. Considerable research is available to anyone on-line, to show that exercise reduces the level of leptin in the blood, and the reduction is proportional to the amount of exercise. Leptin is well known to be a theoretical factor in reducing obesity; unfortunately it has undesirable effects as well such as stimulating the progression of PC. It has a particularly bad effect on the growth of hormone-resistant PC. A good reference on the properties of leptin is the article by LaCava et al., 2003.

Insulin has been shown to be strongly implicated in the development and progression of PC (see also in Chapter 4, Nutrition). An excellent review of the role of exercise in this context is to be found in the *Prostate Cancer Foundation Guide 2009* entitled 'Nutrition, Exercise and Prostate Cancer'.

As mentioned above, exercise stimulates endorphins producing a sense of well-being and a positive outlook. This is why exercise is recommended for people suffering from anxiety and depression in general, but it would seem particularly appropriate in cancer patients also for its general health benefits. It should be noted that, should a man opt for treatment with androgen blockade, depression is one of the fairly common side effects along with tendency to obesity, high blood pressure and osteoporosis. All of these conditions benefit from exercise.

- Exercise also decreases blood sugar and triglyceride levels in the blood
- Decreases the risk of blood clots
- Decreases body fat, especially round the belly which is very important in PC
- Increases metabolism
- Boosts the immune system.

Q. You read about exercise being important, but what sort and how much?

A. For PC patients, Dr Dean Ornish recommends regular, moderate exercise. Browsing through his Preventive Medicine Research Institute website, the patient can follow his approach in detail.

Following is an excerpt: 'The comprehensive lifestyle change program encourages participants to exercise aerobically a minimum of 30 minutes a day or for an hour every other day for a total of 3-5 hours of aerobic exercise per week. More intense exercise is allowed if medically appropriate and if desired by the participant. Resistive or strength training exercise is also crucial to maintaining health. If medically appropriate, participants are also encouraged to engage in strength training exercise 2-3 times per week.'

My wife and I used to exercise by walking, but getting caught in the rain dampened our spirits for that. We then played tennis, but had to drive quite a distance to the courts. We bought a 'strider' which is similar to a tread-mill, but even with a TV set to watch we found the process a bit boring.

We eventually discovered table-tennis, and this is a game which should suit everyone, so long as there is a partner available. Weather is not an issue. Even the standard size table is not necessary – a standard dining table could be made to do though the game would be less vigorous than we now play. Age should not be a barrier. It would be possible to play even from a wheel chair.

Table tennis is not only wonderful exercise, but it is wonderful fun as well. It sharpens up the reflexes and the mind and can be done in two or three sessions a day during any spare moments.

The trampoline offers another fun mode of exercise. Cycling, golf and all the other activities which may be suitable for the individual should be searched out. Use the stairs instead of taking the lift! Some forms of yoga and modified callisthenics may be suitable and can provide adequate aerobic activity.

Then there is 'resistance' or strength exercise for those unable to move about much. This may involve weight lifting or pushing or pulling against a load in some way, such as the spring-loaded devices with pulleys which feature in TV commercials. With a little ingenuity of course, we can make our own 'weights' to lift.

Professor Sali has this to say about exercise:

Exercise can improve immunity, reduce stress and depression, and increase exposure to sunlight, all of which could increase protection against prostate cancer. Some evidence indicates that physical activity can reduce the chance of developing prostate cancer and may even slow the progression of the disease.Resistance exercise in men receiving androgen-deprivation therapy for prostate cancer reduces fatigue and improves quality of life and muscular fitness. It is possible that resistance exercise may also influence loss of bone mass caused by androgen-deprivation therapy.

SUMMARY

The Take-Home Message is, you don't need to have a six-pack abdomen, but you do need to be lean and tough!

Think hard and be guided wisely about an exercise regime. It should not be exhausting, but you should sweat a little and raise your pulse, and you should feel great after each session. For my wife and me, vigorous table tennis does it. Plus walking and having fun with the dog. After all that exercise you should sleep 'like a top' at night.

7
Treatment options and new initiatives

Although all men, once diagnosed, probably follow a similar thinking path regarding their immediate future, I shall give the results of my own questioning about the way forward. For the reader, your own doctor is the one to do this, but you may find it of some interest and be able to identify with the various possible avenues as I found them. Being a medical scientist and a Type A personality, my investigations were fairly thorough.

Q. What was your first practical reaction to being diagnosed?

A. My first reaction was 'cut it out completely'. It seemed to me that removing the tumour burden had to be a real plus, and this common reaction or intuition is well founded, because no matter which therapy is chosen, 'de-bulking' of the primary tumour is going to help (Swanson G et al., 2006; Myers, (a) 2007, p51.) For each one of us, it's a matter of careful consideration of all options with the help of our medical team.

It's a case of finding the least aggressive and most appropriate procedure. There are now so many possible interventions that age is probably no longer a barrier (see following questions). So if you propose to live beyond a few more years and if you are intermediate risk or higher, de-bulking may be the path to follow.

What had transpired in the minutes after being informed that I had prostate cancer was a total blur. I couldn't remember what else the urologist had said. I do remember thinking even at this stage, 'This could be a mistake – pathologists are only human and biopsies have been misread before. We'll get a second opinion.'

My wife and I read up everything we could. There was of course open surgery called radical prostatectomy with which everyone was fairly familiar. In good hands it achieved good results – apparently between 70% and 80% of men were still free of the cancer 10 years after the operation.

The side effects were also well known. The possibility of urinary incontinence and probability of erectile dysfunction or impotence, and no return of the ejaculate. The first two conditions generally improve over time, but we had serious reservations about the procedure because of the increased risks with my age. We therefore decided to explore all other options. The urologist is the one to flesh out details of the actual procedures for you and will explain terms like the optional retropubic or transperineal approach to the prostate, 'positive margins' and so on.

Q. What about this so-called 'key-hole' or 'minimally invasive' surgery?

A. In key-hole – or laparoscopic – prostatectomy, the surgeon operates through instruments placed through the abdominal wall into the abdominal cavity or retro-pubic space, generally via six small incisions, with an 'endoscope' or thin telescope to look through. The procedure is more patient-friendly in the sense that recovery is generally quicker than with open surgery, though it may take longer. There may be less blood loss and 'nerve-sparing' or protection of the erectile nerves as indicated, can be done just as with the open method.

Results appear to be approaching the 'Gold Standard' set by years of experience and research, as achieved for open radical prostatectomy. It is, however, a more difficult and challenging operation with few exponents, compared with open surgery and therefore may not be readily available in Australia.

Q. Then there is 'robotic surgery'. How is this different from the key-hole variety and what sort of results do they get?

A. In robotic surgery, the surgeon operates on the patient while sitting at a console with electronic links to the patient. He/she operates using instruments placed into the abdominal cavity as with key-hole surgery but those instruments are now under the control of the robotic slave. The telescope relays the real-time '3D video' out to the console. Magnification is provided and a sophisticated gearing system allows relatively large movements by the operator, to achieve tiny movements inside the patient, for dissection, nerve bundle identification, removal of the prostate specimen and finally visually accurate, re-anastomosis (surgical joining) of the urethra to the bladder. An associate surgeon and scrub sister are also involved in the operation, both being in direct contact and concurrently operating on the patient.

This technology is not yet readily available in the public hospital system in Australia, but is available in the private health sector at variable cost, depending on one's health insurance cover. There is minimal blood loss, optimum erectile nerve protection and directed, accurate anastomotic visualisation with this method.

The hospital stay is of two days duration and like all radical prostatectomy techniques, a urethral catheter is required during the anastomotic healing process. As with the previous answer, we found the cost prohibitive unless no other option could be found.

Q. A man in the local support group had cryosurgery. What is that?

A. This method is an adaption of old technology and applicable to patients not suitable for the more established treatments. See below under 'promising treatment modalities'.

Q. Another of the group had HIFU. Is this like cryosurgery?

A. No, in this procedure a probe is inserted into the rectum and High Intensity Focused Ultrasound (HIFU) waves are directed at the prostate to destroy the tissue. It is a treatment selected when surgery and/or irradiation are not suitable or accepted. It can be repeated and has some exponents in Australia. The main background work in this field has been done in China and Japan. The potential side effects are again impotence, incontinence and urethral strictures, as well as fistula formation Once again, a relatively new treatment to Australia. Also not covered by Medicare.

Q. Did you consider radiation?

A. Yes, in fact I was enrolled in an External Beam Radiation Therapy (EBRT) program which kills cancer cells by X-rays. Nomograms – which enable reasonably accurate assessment of risk for a given patient's test results – were explained by the radiation oncologist. We went through the preliminaries and had organised my trips to the hospital for five days a week over seven weeks.

In terms of EBRT outcomes according to most surveys, after 8 years the survival rate ranges from 70% to 80% for low risk patients to about 40% for high risk patients. Short term side effects were likely to consist of diarrhoea, skin discomfort and tiredness. Longer term, impotence was likely to be a problem with bowel incontinence less of a problem.

For some months we had been thinking of getting second opinions about various aspects of my PC ranging from the pathology report to laser procedures which a medical friend had mentioned. My urologist went on holidays, and at about this time I began to develop increasing obstructive urinary symptoms, high residual urine volumes which culminated in urinary retention. There were also back pressure effects on my renal function. The on-call urologist at the hospital advised TransUrethral Resection of the Prostate (TURP) since I had only one kidney, having had the other removed many years ago.

This new urologist, Donald Murphy MD, FRACS now became our 'second opinion' and we have stayed with him ever since on our journey. His guidance, both from the PC point of view and in the 'urological' side of this book, has been invaluable.

Q. Did you think about brachytherapy at all?

A. Brachytherapy is a term used when the radiation source itself is placed inside the area being treated. It is performed in one of two ways, either one-off permanent seed implants, or removable 'interstitial' iridium wires over a period of days. I would have liked to have used the former because it does not have the weeks of visits to the hospital, requiring just an overnight stay. Radioactive seeds are implanted through the perineum (between the anus and the scrotum) into the cancerous areas of prostate tissue, where they release X-rays over a long period. Five-year cancer-free figures of about 80% are usually quoted. Side effects can include bladder and urine flow problems which are usually temporary. Impotence and bowel issues are fairly common, but once again should resolve.

In my case, having had a TURP precluded my having brachytherapy because so much tissue had been removed that the radioactive seeds may not 'hold' in the prostate.

Q. Did you consider any other treatments?

A. We thought about pharmacological androgen ablation therapy which is dealt with in some detail in Chapter 5 and Appendix 3. The severe side effects did not appeal. In any case, this mode of treatment is usually reserved for men who fail one of the other primary interventions and/or have aggressive, widespread cancer. A Urologist or medical oncologist are the usual specialists to advise on this approach.

Dr Robert Leibowitz, a medical oncologist specialising in prostate cancer in the US, has a unique approach to androgen ablation or blockade. The usual modes of blockade are either intermittent or continuous, and there is considerable literature on each. Leibowitz and his colleague, Dr Charles Myers mentioned above, use 13 months of aggressive blockade. The blockade is then stopped permanently, to be followed only by on-going maintenance with either Proscar or Avodart. Both of these compounds inhibit the enzyme (5-alpha-reductase) which turns testosterone into dihydrotestosterone or DHT. This androgen is much more potent than testosterone.

Over a period of more than ten years, these oncologists have achieved quite remarkable results with their approach (Tucker & Leibowitz, 2005; Leibowitz, 2008). They consider the 13 months necessary to ensure lasting 'kill' of the cancer cells, though the men suffer the severe side-effects without the on-and-off 'holiday' which intermittent therapy offers. Nevertheless, long term follow-up shows excellent PSA control and more importantly, a disease-specific survival rate of better than 99%.

Could it be that using Prostasol or Quercetin Plus instead of the unpleasant hormonal blockade might be a better approach? After all, these herbal treatments also reduce PSA to effectively undetectable levels as discussed above in Chapter 5, but without the unpleasant side-effects. See more on a possible alternative regime in Appendix 3.

Because of my involvement in medical research into prostate cancer, I was aware of other experimental procedures and methods being trialled. For example, proton beam radiation therapy involves targeting the cancer with a stream of high energy protons. Of these modalities, however, there was nothing which appealed and was practical. So after consultation with the medical advisors we had now built up – and after reading research by Professor Dean Ornish and others, also discussed in Chapters 4 and 5 – we decided to 'go natural'.

'Going natural' has meant proactive surveillance with Mind-body Medicine, meditation, nutrition and supplements and exercise, together with fairly regular assessment of my PSA and other status parameters. With regard to Prostasol (or Quercetin Plus), it is a powerful supplement and perhaps should be used only if and when the PC shows signs of 'taking off', as indicated by the PSA and other investigations already discussed.

One of the arguments for the appropriate embracing of Active Surveillance, is that it ideally suits pro-active control of the PC chronic condition, which for many men has little impact on their life. It is therefore understandable that men with low risk disease – or older men with intermediate risk disease – might prefer not to embark on other treatments which can be debilitating. Novel management and new treatments are developing as discussed in this chapter and eventually a definitive cure/control for PC will be found.

Q. What promising treatment modalities are available now or 'in the pipeline'?

A. New approaches and breakthroughs appear in the medical literature on a regular basis. Following are some of the more recent ones:
It was reported in *Medical News Today*, 11th February 2010, that urologists and scientists at Queen's University and Kingston General Hospital have been using very low-dose nitroglycerin patches to treat recurring prostate cancer. Preliminary results show its potential to halt the disease.

A new antibody against prostate cancer cells has recently been developed to seek out and kill the cells wherever they are in the body. Using mice as a model, the Philadelphia investigators found that the new antibody named F77, effectively bonded to and destroyed 97% of cancer cells, and 85% of metastasized cancer cells. It even recognised androgen-resistant cancer cells. The antibody did not impact on normal cells. This result holds out great hope for PC treatment in humans. Reported in Uro Today, 7th January, 2010.

A form of cryo-surgery has made headlines recently with regard to prostate cancer. Cryosurgery involves freezing of the organ or part of it. It was reported in *Medical News Today* on 10th March, 2009, that this minimally invasive interventional radiology treatment for prostate cancer is as effective as surgery in destroying diseased tumors. It can be considered a first-line treatment for patients of all risk levels.

Data show that cryoablation is as good for prostate cancer control as any other treatment – including surgery, radiation and hormone therapy – but it is less invasive and traumatic for patients, preserves sexual and urinary function and has no major complications. Interventional radiologists tailor treatment to each patient's disease. "Instead of removing the entire prostate, or freezing the entire prostate or using radiation on the entire prostate, interventional radiologists can find out where the cancer is and just destroy the cancer," said study author Gary M. Onik, M.D., interventional radiologist and director of the Center for Safer Prostate Cancer Therapy in Orlando, Fla. The procedure uses a special 3-D mapping biopsy for determining the extent of prostate cancer. The question remains as to whether any mapping – 'special' or not – is accurate.

"There is no question that we can eradicate prostate cancer (when that cancer has not spread to other parts of the body) by freezing it and that there is a better way to 'map' the disease," said Onik. "Recently the American Urological Association issued a best practice statement that indicated that cryotherapy is an option for men who have clinically organ-confined prostate cancer of any grade with negative metastatic evaluation. Since this interventional treatment is not widely known to doctors and patients, individuals will need to pursue it on their own," he added.

My urologist reminded me that Cryotherapy for prostate treatment has been promoted for many years, but it has not stood the test of time. He argues this point, "taking into account efficacy, equipment costs, side effects, 'ice-ball' penetration and incomplete margin treatment, because of the 'heat sink' associated with the prostatic venous system. The side effects include fistulas to bowel, urethral strictures, urinary incontinence and bladder damage." He acknowledges that things may have changed in recent times with further research.

Researchers at Children's Hospital Boston have isolated a potent inhibitor of tumor metastasis made by tumor cells, one that could potentially be harnessed as a cancer treatment. Their findings were published in the online Early Edition of the *Proceedings of the National Academy of Sciences* during the week of June 22, 2009.

Metastasis – the migration of cancer cells to other parts of the body – is one of the leading causes of death from cancer, and there is no approved therapy for inhibiting or treating metastases. Randoph S. Watnick, PhD, an assistant professor in the Vascular Biology Program at Children's, has been finding that metastatic tumors prepare landing places in distant organs for their metastases, by secreting certain proteins that encourage tumor growth and attract feeder blood vessels. Now, he and his colleagues show that non-metastatic tumors secrete a protein called prosaposin – which inhibits metastasis by causing production of factors that block the growth of blood vessels.

When the researchers injected mice with tumor cells that were known to be highly metastatic, but to which they had added prosaposin, lung metastases were reduced by 80% and lymph node metastases were completely eliminated, and survival time was significantly increased. Conversely, when they suppressed prosaposin expression in tumor cells, they saw more metastases. When prosaposin was directly injected into mice that had also received an injection of tumor cells, the tumor cells formed virtually no metastases in the lung, or, if they did, formed much smaller colonies.

Watnick and colleagues also demonstrated that prosaposin stimulates activity of the well-known tumor suppressor p53 in the connective tissue surrounding the tumor.

Irreversible electroporation (IRE) This is commonly called 'nano-knife'. It is radiologically guided microsurgery and causes cell death by impacting the cell membranes with electrical pulses in targeted tissue, sparing nerves, blood vessels, lymphatic system and other nearby delicate structures. While quite a new procedure in this context – though the process has been employed to deliver drugs for some time – IRE has recently been used successfully in human liver, kidney and prostate cancers J.Urol. 2008 October. E-pub ahead of print. PubMed Abs: 18951581. Dr Gary Onik from Florida Hospital, a pioneer in the development of the procedure, has successfully treated 17 PC patients with IRE (personal communication).

A new study shows that an alpha-particle emitting radiopeptide – radioactive material bound to a synthetic peptide, a component of protein – is effective for treating prostate cancer in mice, it was reported in *Science Daily*, June 25, 2009. The results could eventually result in a significant breakthrough in prostate cancer treatment, especially for patients whose cancer recurs after the prostate is removed.

This novel form of treatment has the potential to target and destroy cancer cells with minimal damage to surrounding healthy tissue," said Damian Wild, University

Hospital Basel, Basel, Switzerland, lead author of the study. "Eventually, this therapy could give hope to some of the hardest-to-treat prostate cancer patients and also could be applied to other types of cancer."

MRI-guided transurethral ultrasound The treatment is minimally invasive and takes less than 30 minutes. Heat from focused ultrasound is applied via the urethra – the penis in the male – precisely to the tumour from inside, thus sparing the non-cancerous tissues around the prostate essential for healthy urinary, bowel and sexual function (*Medical News Today*, September 2008).

Once again, my urologist Donald Murphy, commented that, "Prostate cancer, according to the McNeal model is more important when it is in the peripheral zone, not the central zone. This treatment as discussed above is maximized to the central, peri-urethral areas." What this means is that the region where most prostate cancer cells usually reside, is not getting the full effect of this treatment. For more information on the McNeal model, see Glossary.

Abiraterone Up to 80% of patients with aggressive and previously drug-resistant PC could be treated with this drug which was discovered at the Institute of Cancer Research and the Royal Marsden Hospital in the UK. Clinical effects achieved in patients included evidence of PSA falls and tumour shrinkage in 70 to 80% of patients as demonstrated by CAT scans, MRI and bone scans. All this with few side effects (*Medical News Today*, 29 July 2008). See Appendix 3 for more information.

The use of ***Heat activated liposomes*** allows the direct delivery of chemotherapeutic drugs directly to a target tissue such as the prostate. Roswell Park Cancer Institute researchers have developed this procedure to offset the severe toxicities associated with conventional chemotherapy. In animal studies, they found that the heat activated liposomes resulted in 'profound biological effects on the gland with no apparent safety concerns such as urinary tract problems'.

Metformin is an anti-diabetic medication. Recent epidemiological studies have demonstrated that this drug has anti-cancer effects and may be useful in the treatment of PC. It has been established that metformin exerts its anti-tumoural effect by blocking the cell cycle (Ben Sahra et al., 2008).

How to sift out which prostate cancers are going to be 'tigers' (aggressive) and which are going to be 'pussy cats' (harmless)! Scientists from the Institute of Cancer Research and The Royal Marsden Hospital in the UK, won the 2008 Medical Futures Innovation Award for coming up with a method to do just that! The idea is to use 'diffusion weighted' Magnetic Resonance Imaging to differentiate between the two and so dramatically improve the way PC is diagnosed. By extension, the procedure could be used to monitor the status or progress of a cancer whether under therapy or Active Surveillance.

Sunflower seeds contain a mini-protein which could be the key to stopping tumours from spreading in PC patients. Queensland University of Technology scientists are interested in this protein particularly for patients who relapse. The focus of their research is to stop the disease from spreading, since it not the prostate tumour which kills, but metastases formed when the cancer cells escape from the prostate. Reported in *Medical News Today*, May 2, 2008.

Vaccines There are quite a few being developed, such as one which has been proven to identify and destroy PC cells in animals with first human trials now underway. The vaccine uses synthetic proteins which mimic the largest molecule on the cancer. This in turn stimulates the patient's immune system to identify cancerous cells and instruct other cells to destroy them. The research is being conducted by scientists at the Mater Medical Research Institute in Brisbane, Australia.

Another similar product is Vakzine which is being used with promising results for patients with advanced, hormone-resistant PC. The study was carried out at the Institute for Experimental Oncology, Hanover, Germany in 2007.

Scientists at Melbourne's Burnet Institute have developed a potential new treatment for patients with prostate cancer. It was reported in Science Alert (Australia and New Zealand) on February 9th 2009 that the group has produced a specific antibody to a unique tumour marker for the treatment of prostate cancer. The monoclonal antibody is directed at cancer-producing cells carrying the specific molecule known as PIM-1, which is responsible for cell survival, proliferation and differentiation.

University of Southern California scientists have developed a vaccine which turns PC in mice into a chronic, manageable disease. They prevented the development of cancer in 90% of mice genetically predestined to develop the disease, by confronting the immune system in two different ways to force a strong response against a prostate cancer cell antigen. News release February 1st 2008, USC website www.aacr.org

In a Phase 11 trial, 27 patients with metastatic hormone refractory PC were treated with Trovax. All available patients experienced robust antibody response against the targeted tumour antigen. 83% of these 'very difficult' patients experienced disease stabilization (*Medical News Today*, March 26, 2008).

In a recent set of trials by Cell Genesys, immunotherapy with 'GVAX' resulted in a statistically significant increase in median PSA doubling time. 84% of patients with recurrent PC experienced a decline in PSA slope and the treatment was well tolerated. This was reported in the April 11th 2008 edition of the Pharmaceutical Drugs Information on-line site, Drugs.com.

Provenge is like a vaccine, wherein immune cells from the patient are treated so that they go back and educate the body's other immune cells to attack the cancer cells The compound was developed at Mary Crowley Medical Research Centre, Dallas Texas in 2007. In a clinical study, the therapy tripled survival rates in men who received it with minimal side effects.

Nano-medicine means engineering compounds on a molecular or atomic scale to be delivered directly to targeted sites of PC. For example, at Weill Cornell Medical College they have developed an antibody against the best PC cell surface target known. The aim is to target this antigen on blood vessels to directly attack a tumour's blood supply without affecting normal vessels.

Other

– Researchers at Adelaide University's Roma Mitchell Cancer Research Laboratories have discovered that by using existing PC cancer drugs in combination with new drugs at lower doses, they can inhibit cancer cell proliferation by more than 10-fold, hopefully making current treatments much more effective and causing fewer side effects. The new therapy will now be tested in patients with advanced PC (*Medical News Today*, July 31st 2008).

– At Yale Cancer Centre, it has been found in a clinical research study that phenoxodiol – a synthetic version of the soy component genistein, see Chapter 5 – had a dose-dependant anti-tumour effect in men with refractory PC. The trial was designed to end after 24 weeks of treatment but was extended to 90 weeks because of the unexpected prolongation of time to progression in some patients. No toxicities were reported. Earlier study showed that phenoxodiol delays disease progression (*Medical News Today*, June 4th, 2008).

– In the Proceedings of the National Academy of Science (2007; vol.104: 1331–1336) it was reported that an androgen receptor decoy molecule has been discovered which decreased serum PSA in all test mice by more than 90%, whereas PSA began to rise rapidly in control mice. Special biochemical staining of tumours showed decreased proliferation in the decoy tumours. Further analysis showed that reduced tumour growth was due to increased cell death in addition to decreased proliferation. The decoy worked in both androgen-dependant and androgen-independent tumours.

– A chemical called noscapine promises to be an effective non-toxic treatment for prostate cancer (published in December issue of the European journal Anticancer Research, 2008). This compound is an ingredient in certain cough mixtures so its safety profile has been well established. The researchers point out that it is without side effects, and that the dose required to effectively treat prostate cancer in the animal model which they used was also safe. The next step is to do trials in humans.

– A key piece to the pin-pointing of aggressive prostate cancer has been found by scientists at the University of Michigan, Ann Arbor. They found that urine levels of a particular amino acid called sarcosine can indicate whether a man has aggressive or benign PC. Reported in *WebMD Health News*, February 11th, 2009.

– Further new developments are gene therapy to stop the advance of diseases, monoclonal antibodies that zap cancer cells throughout the body, drugs that choke off the blood supply to tumours, just to name a few mentioned in the Johns Hopkins University *Bulletin*, October 2008.

– Researchers at North Carolina State University have successfully modified a common plant virus to deliver drugs only to specific cells inside the human body, without affecting surrounding tissue. These tiny nano-particles or "smart bombs" – each one thousands of times smaller than the width of a human hair – could lead to more effective chemotherapy treatments with greatly reduced, or even eliminated, side effects. Reported in *DailyTech* (Science) February 13th, 2009.

– A medical diagnostic company (Miraculins Inc USA) has developed a urine test which, coupled with a particular PSA test, considerably improves the blood marker in PC patients. This means that potentially aggressive PC can be differentiated from 'harmless' PC much more readily, thus sparing biopsies and possibly unnecessary treatment. This was reported in *Medical News Today*, February 12th, 2009.

– Another biomarker for the dangerous form of PC has been discovered by Wake Forest University School of Medicine. This too should provide some direction for men diagnosed with PC about whether their cancer is likely to be life-threatening (*Medical News Today*, February 13th, 2009).

– A measles virus may prove to be effective as a treatment for patients with advanced PC, according to a report in *The Prostate*, January 22nd, 2009.

– Scientists at Oxford University have tamed a virus so that it attacks and destroys cancer cells but does not harm healthy cells. They determined how to produce replication-competent viruses with key toxicities removed, providing a new platform for development of improved cancer treatments and better vaccines for a broad range of viral diseases. (*Science Daily*, May 25th 2009).

– Photo Dynamic Therapy (PDT) is a rediscovery of an old procedure. The first generation model was Russian. The Chinese have taken this technology up a few notches and now the National Institute for Integrative Medicine is studying its potential application here. Basically, in PDT the patient ingests a 'photosensitizing' medication which is taken up only by cancer cells. A specific type of light (laser) is then 'shone' into the body and it activates the medication, to produce a form of oxygen which is lethal to whatever cells have taken it up.

This procedure is pain-free, requires no hospitalisation, and has been shown to act effectively on solid tumours and is likely to be useful in the treatment of prostate cancer. Further research will establish its long term future as a novel therapy for the condition. More information is available on the National Cancer Institute Fact Sheet.

Obviously there is a huge push going on in the world of medical science, to differentiate dangerous from harmless PC and to stop it, or at least to control it. Heartening news for those of us who have the condition and for those of us who may get it! Almost every week this sort of innovative research is reported, and this should be further grounds for optimism . . .

The hope is that the reader may have found much in this book to make him feel less anxious and more positive.

Life lived 'in the present moment' is far more enjoyable – whatever may be ahead – than wallowing in the past or agonising about the future. We can address issues as they arise, even plan to the extent that prudence requires, but then we should drop it. Return to the present, do something constructive. Maybe play tennis or go shopping with your spouse or your partner or your friend, or go for a run with your dog, or perhaps just sit in the garden and watch the bees . . .

Finally, develop the skill of deep meditation. Gently and without stress, immerse yourself in the Big Picture. Seek and you will find Truth, and the Truth will set you free . . .

SUMMARY

The Take-Home Message is, there are excellent existing treatment options, and powerful initiatives just round the corner. Prostate cancer will be beaten!

Your carefully chosen team will advise you. All I can add is, give the treatment of choice your best shot and embrace Active Surveillance no matter what. Be optimistic, but of course no-one lives forever, so don't aim for that – perhaps it is written that you will die of old age!

My wife's and my personal belief is that all this is in better Hands than ours, and the best is yet to come!

Appendix 1

Further thoughts on Prostate Cancer

Its Origins and Development

With Notes by Mr Donald Murphy MBBS, MD, FRACS.

Prostate cancer as a disease has a wide spectrum of presentations. The condition has as its basic aetiology, an imbalance of genetic expression and contributing environmental factors. The latter are intimately related to testosterone factors, as well as external environmental influences, including dietary intake.

Huggins and Hodges in 1941 published literature linking prostate cancer to testosterone, and they initiated the treatment of surgical removal of the testicles for advanced cases. In 1966 Charles Huggins was co-awarded the Nobel Prize for medicine for this work.

Genetic research in prostate cancer is ongoing and will, I believe, in the future direct methods of prostate cancer diagnosis and care.

As discussed in this book, dietary factors also have a very important part to play.

The lowest incidence of prostate cancer occurs in the adult males of the northern Japanese islands, where Soya bean products and fish are in their staple diet. Direct Japanese relatives of these males, living in America and on a stable American diet, have a much higher incidence of prostate cancer, equal to the general American population. In contrast, the Afro-American adult male population in the same environment has the highest incidence of prostate cancer in the world.

To make the diagnosis of prostate cancer, three things are involved: firstly a PSA blood test, secondly an internal digital rectal examination (DRE) to assess the prostate characteristics and thirdly a prostate tissue biopsy. The biopsy is carried out because of an elevation in the PSA level and/or an abnormality, on the rectal prostate examination. Needless to say a patient can have a normal PSA and rectal examination and still have microscopic prostate cancer. The place of continuing surveillance for such a patient is suggested, as appropriate ongoing medical care.

Morbidity and mortality are important factors to be remembered when discussing prostate cancer treatments. The incidence of prostate cancer, as related in this book effects up to 80% of 90 year males. The disease at this older age may be indolent, asymptomatic and not needing any medical intervention.

The question is, who needs interventional aggressive treatment, if this diagnosis is made? The exact answer to that question is unknown and at this time of knowledge, patients are treated on a case-by-case decision, involving informed consent with the patient's age and co-morbidities as relevant factors.

On the other hand prostate cancer may follow an aggressive course and be fatal, particularly for younger males. Under these circumstances the histological features of the prostate cancer are usually of high-grade, with high Gleason scores.

Overall, however, any aggressive interventional treatment for prostate cancer should be aimed at making a difference to the person's life in 10 to 12 years. This is the predicted time of prostate cancer natural progression, relating to the indolent nature of the majority of prostate cancers.

Treatment options for prostate cancer with intent to cure are primarily surgery and irradiation. Other treatments, such as hormone therapy, chemotherapy, cryosurgery, HIFU also exist, depending on the clinical scenario and desired outcome.

The age and underlying health of the man, the presence/extent of metastasis, appearance under the microscope or Gleason score, and response of the cancer to initial treatment are important in determining the prognosis of this disease and the treatment options.

The decision whether or not to treat localised prostate cancer (a tumor that is contained within the prostate) with curative intent is a patient decision, considering the expected beneficial and harmful effects, in terms of patient survival and quality of life.

In Chapter 7 we reviewed Treatment Options and New Initiatives. Now it might be helpful to look briefly at other research being done with prospects perhaps further down the track.

Donald Murphy suggested to me one day that I look into the embryology of prostate cancer – that means, could a future key to understanding prostate cancer therapy have origins in the womb? He reminded me of the 'descent of the testicles' which happens *in-utero* from about weeks thirty two to thirty six weeks of male foetal development. A surge in testosterone accompanies this descent. By the time of full term delivery, this surge is turned off.

The testosterone increase is also associated with neonatal prostate growth and an elevated PSA test. Apoptosis (planned cell death) occurs in this neonatal prostatic tissue, usually by three months of age, as a result of the turn off of the testosterone source. At puberty, with reactivation of testosterone release, the prostate again grows to perform its planned functions for future fertility. Future research will reveal if the off switch can again be activated as possible benign and malignant prostate treatments.

Our research into the above matter has identified the involvement of such diverse factors as Mullerian Inhibiting Substance, stem cells and foetal endocrinology. It may be helpful to offer a very basic and brief explanation of these concepts.

Mullerian Inhibiting Substance is a product of the embryonic testis. It 'turns off' the pathway towards female development. Recent thinking is that it may have a wider role in the development of prostate cancer. Scientists at Harvard Medical School are studying the way in which this substance regulates androgen-induced gene expression in prostate cancer cells.

Stem cells are so-called 'master cells' which can develop into any or all of the cell types in the body. A search has been on to identify the stem cells of prostate cancer tissue, with a view to modifying them. Recent reports suggest that this aim has been met, although it is not within the scope of our book to go further into the subject. Sufficient to say that some laboratories such as the Yorkshire Cancer Research Unit at the University of York, are already using putative PC stem cells to investigate the PC tumorigenic process.

With regard to foetal endocrinology or hormones, many laboratories have been trying to unravel the relationship between the oestrogens and the androgens and their role in early prostate development. For example, it seems that high levels of oestrogens induce prostate cancer but only in combination with high levels of androgens.

Gail Risbridger and her team at the Centre for Urological Research at Monash Institute of Medical Research, Melbourne, are addressing these sorts of questions. Can such an imbalance occur in the foetus? Could early prostate development be associated with later-life prostate disease? Oestrogen acts via two receptor types, alpha and beta, and it is known that imbalance between the two is involved in the development of prostate cancer. Could we manipulate these forms to influence the outcome?

Somewhere in all this may lie the definitive answer to our questions.

Appendix 2

The support person's perspective

by Elizabeth Meade

I was very pleased to be asked to contribute this section. These are the things I found hard to handle when my husband was diagnosed with prostate cancer:

The waiting room. In our GP's waiting room there are men, women and children of all ages. Perhaps even babies. There is a fairly friendly atmosphere with lots of movement. Doctors popping their heads in and staff ushering patients to and fro. When Brian was first diagnosed, in the urologist's waiting room there were usually just a few elderly men looking frail and unwell. The atmosphere can be depressing.

When the doctor first told us that it was prostate cancer, I felt shock and unbelief. I know my husband felt the same but it must have been much deeper. All my attention and concern was for him, however. It was only later that I reflected on how this might impact my life.

None of the doctors or specialists we saw at this time – GPs, surgeon, radiation oncologists – asked as to how all this was affecting me. We decided to get a second opinion. The new urologist (Donald Murphy) restored our confidence that things weren't so dismal considering the possible 10 to 12 year, natural PC history. On his suggestion, we could first try natural therapies including for example Epilobium and soy products instead of aggressive interventions. An Active Surveillance programme was appropriate for Brian, at 74 years of age. We were encouraged, together, to further research PC disease. Later, the Integrative Medicine specialist (Avni Sali) also strongly encouraged the 'partnership' approach. We would share everything by what he called 'unloading' it all, as well as everything else from massage to going to the movies together.

My early reactions were of pity for my husband. Then there was worry and fear of the possible consequences. Is he likely to die from this? I then put thoughts about my own future aside and focused on what I could do to help. I was determined to spend myself for him no matter what it took. We would raise any money if there were some way to cure him.

I had sleepless nights. There were periods of depression and anxiety. Daytime chores became hum-drum as we tried to come to grips with this new reality in our lives. Our feelings were unreal as we stumbled from one examination to another. Then there were all the blood tests, scans and other procedures in between.

Some of the specialists gave us the statistics in a fairly matter-of-fact way. I felt like the wife of a statistic. Waiting for results was painfully slow. More visits to the specialists for explanations and alternatives. In fact we had the advantage that my husband was doing medical research and we were pretty well informed. Even so, during the waiting there was a feeling of helplessness.

Decision time. After discussions with Professor Sali and the urologist Donald Murphy, and taking everything into account, we decided to forego aggressive interventions and take on Active Surveillance. Even though my husband was 'intermediate' level prostate cancer.

My husband decided to go on a vegetarian diet as suggested by the scientific literature. This meant I had to cook two different meals or eat what he ate. I decided to do the latter and eat the same. He needed daily fresh vegetable juice so we bought a juicer. He could not have 'dairy' so we did without butter, cheese and cow's milk. Unfortunately we over-did the diet thing and we both lost too much weight.

My husband had reservations about my writing the next bit. But I insisted. We rekindled our belief in a 'Higher being' as the literature calls it. Our rejuvenated Faith was an enormous help and we have continued to work on it. Our love for each other has grown stronger and stronger during this period of trial.

My husband's PSA has come down and he is very fit and happy. We are fortunate to be able to assist 'the cause' with medical research, but most men can help in some way, whether financially or volunteering via support groups, or perhaps praying for others.

Finally, it is good to see that 'carers' in general are slowly being recognised by governments and aid agencies in the western world. The support persons of prostate cancer sufferers, whether spouses or not, also need recognition and help. More from a psychological point of view than anything else such as money or labour saving devices. I especially feel for those who have worse cases to support than I do. May your journey together be successful in the very best sense of the word.

Author's note to Appendix 2: When first diagnosed with PC, I tended to feel sorry for myself. It seemed natural to let my wife worry about me, fuss over me and get on with the new diet and whatever was required to get me well.

It took longer than it should have, for me to realise how deeply my wife was suffering too. I don't think there is any argument that women are by nature more self-sacrificing than men, so it is something we could easily take for granted. It seems to me that to avoid this happening, we men have to forget our own pre-occupation to a very large extent and concern ourselves with the needs and well being of our 'support person'. Indeed, doing this will have a therapeutic effect on everyone involved.

Appendix 3

Notes for the Advanced Reader

Abbreviations in molecular biology literature are puzzling to the reader who is not an expert. The abbreviations usually consist of three or four letters, and sometimes it is clear as to what the abbreviation means but quite often not. Who would ever guess that *SMAC* stands for *S*econdary *M*itochondrial-derived *A*ctivator of *C*aspase?

This Appendix is for the reader who is moderately well informed, to the degree that he/she is not afraid of scientific material which is a bit challenging if it helps to paint a clearer picture. Such a reader may choose to follow up the meaning of the abbreviations used, but this is not necessary to gain a fair understanding. From my experience, most PC sufferers are sufficiently motivated to read anything which looks helpful, and many are quite capable of learning from this Appendix.

At support group meetings, there is a natural sharing of knowledge and the medical jargon becomes less frightening when one is part of such a group. The talks by guest pathologists and others also dispel much of the mystique. Many of the men are quite at home talking about Gleason scores, lymph nodes and PSA velocity. Some will even be heard explaining things like endo-rectal MRI or suppressor genes to their attentive but less knowledgeable audience. And this is generally good.

For the reader who does want to know what the abbreviations stand for, he/she will find the web site www.Beelib.com most helpful.

P16. *Klotz criteria.* Good risk PC is defined as a Gleason score of 6 or less, PSA < 10ng/ml, and T1c to T2a (see Glossary for explanation). For men over 70yrs of age, the conditions may be relaxed to allow intermediate-risk PC (that is, Gleason score of 3+4=7).

P22. *PsychoNeuroEndocrinology or PNE.* There is a well researched connection between the endocrine and immune systems.

Glucocorticoids and catecholamines influence immune cells

Glucocorticoids cause immunosuppression

Anti-inflammatory hormones enhance the organism's response to a stressor.

P32. Suppression of cellular immunity is associated with particular conditions, such as Epstein-Barr (EBV) associated lymphoproliferative diseases in organ transplant patients, and Kaposi's sarcoma and EBV associated B-cell lymphoma in AIDS patients.

P44. *Movement and invasion (after Myers, 2000)* by PC cells is facilitated by the conversion of the fatty acid arachidonic acid to a substance called 12-HETE. Inhibitors of

12-HETE formation are remarkably effective at arresting the movement of human prostate cancer cells.

Patients with tumors able to make 12-HETE have been found much more likely to develop metastatic prostate cancer after radical prostatectomy. Given the ability of 12-HETE to foster cancer cell invasion and new blood vessel formation these findings are hardly surprising.

When arachidonic acid (AA) is acted on by an enzyme called 5-LOX, a metabolite called 5-HETE is formed. This eicosanoid is well established to have serious effects on cancer cell survival, growth and invasion. It can evade the immune system and it promotes generation of new blood vessels for the cancer.

When the formation of 5-HETE is completely blocked, all human prostate cancer cell lines that have been able to be tested, stop growing and die within a few hours. Human prostate cancer cells contain a suicide program waiting to be activated. Hormonal therapy, radiation therapy, and chemotherapy treatments for prostate cancer work by activating this suicide program. None of these treatments cause cancer cell death as rapidly as is seen after blocking 5-HETE formation.

P45. *Arachidonic acid.* This fatty acid can be converted to a chemical PGE2. Human prostate cancer cells produce PGE2 from arachidonic acid. In radical prostatectomy specimens, the cancer produced ten times as much PGE2 as the surrounding normal prostate tissue! PGE2 is very toxic to both natural killer cells and cytotoxic T cells and is one potential mechanism by which prostate cancer defeats the immune system (Myers, 2000).

P49. *Barnard et al.* In their Review (on prostate cancer), they noted that hyperinsulinaemia has been shown to have a direct effect on the liver. There it suppresses the production of sex hormone-binding globulin (SHBG) and insulin-like growth factor-binding proteins 1 and 2 (IGFBP-1, -2) while stimulating the production of insulin-like growth factor 1 (IGF-1).

They observed that men adopting a low-fat diet and daily exercise reduced their levels of serum insulin and IGF-1, while increasing their levels of IGFBP-1 and sex hormone-binding globulin (SHBG).

P51. *Further insights* . . . Further insights into the insulin labyrinth: Linoleic Acid may be changed by an enzyme Delta-6-Desaturase into Gamma Linolenic Acid which may then be changed by another enzyme Elongase into Dihomo Gamma Linolenic Acid (DGLA).

Delta 6-Desaturase is stimulated by Insulin and the more Insulin the more DGLA is preferentially converted into AA, instead of being converted into less harmful products by the other enzyme cyclo-oxygenase-1 (COX-1). Eating oily fish or taking fish-oil supplements which include EPA will reduce the effect of Delta-6-Desaturase.

P59. *PEITC* (phenylethylisothiocyanate) is a constituent of many vegetables, especially brassicas like cabbage and cauliflour. The isothiocyanates are further digested to produce DIM (diindolylmethane), a very important compound in relation to PC. DIM is best delivered via the skin.

P59. *Further information about Brassica vegetables.* An excellent summary of the mechanisms of action are contained in an article by Keck et al., 2004. They discuss detoxification, protection against oxidative stress, tumour growth unhibition and apoptosis altered estrogen metabolism. Sulforaphane and indole-3-carbinol (I3C) both inhibit the AR. They both increase Phase 11 enzymes. They also induce apoptosis in PC cells via Reactive Oxygen Species (ROS) generation. They enhance Fas, the so-called death-receptor. Both enhance p53 and Bax, while stimulating the action of ERK. Both also inhibit Bcl-2 and NFkB.

I3C is a precursor of diindolyl methane (DIM) and it uncouples ER-alpha & ER-beta, increasing the ratio ERbeta/ERalpha which is very good news for PC sufferers. It also depresses the AR.

DIM is a pure AR antagonist which tends to improve the ratio of 2-OH to 16-OH oestrogens. According to Mohammad MR et al. (2007) it reduces the activity of Akt, NF-kB and AR phosphorylation. DIM reduces the expression of AR and PSA. Enhances caspases which are pro-apoptotic. Other actions which are beneficial to PC sufferers, it lowers Bcl-2, BAD, IAP, FLIP, survivin and TNF receptor-associated factor 1. It inhibits the MAPK pathway and upregulates the phosphorylation of Akt. It enhances the TRAIL receptor, increases phosphorylation of B-catenin leading towards apoptosis. DIM is best delivered transdermally since absorption by the intestines is limited.

Phenylethylisothiocyanate or PEITC reduces angiogenesis by stimulating Bax and Bak It stimulates caspase and therefore apoptosis. It down-regulates mutant p53 tumour growth. It is synergistic with curcumin and inhibits NF-kB and PKC.

P60. *Caloric restriction* has a dramatic effect on blood levels of the undesirable compounds leptin, IL-6, CRP and TNF (Myers, 2007 b). Such restriction can easily be overdone, however, so collaboration with medical advisors is important.

P60. *Abiraterone* shows greater than 50% reduction in PSA in 70% of castration-resistant PC patients. Another second-generation anti-androgen which shows real promise in castration-resistant PC is MDV3100, which will soon replace bicalutamide in castration-resistant PC.

P66. *Further information on vitamin D.*
The following properties and actions of this remarkable hormone are from authorities and researchers such as Hollick, M (2007), Khan, M (2004), Matilainen, M et al., 2005.

Reduces growth of PC cells by stimulating differentiation.
Induces cell cycle arrest and apoptosis.
Reduces invasion and adhesion of androgen-independent PC cell lines *in vitro* as well as in xenografts.
Inhibits MMP-9 and cathepsin.
Regulates IGF-BPs and increases PSADT.
It is a potent immuno-modulator.

Given the critical significance of IGFs and the various binding proteins which modulate their action in cancer cells (see Chapter 4), the following functions of vitamin D become of very great importance:

IGFBP1, 3 and 5 are primary target genes for $1{,}25(OH)_2D3$. IGFBPs mediate IGF-independent actions, including the activation of the p21 gene, causing cell cycle arrest or cell death through apoptosis.

P71. *Genistein* from soy inhibits the activation of the nuclear transcription factor, NF-κB and Akt signalling pathway, both of which are known to maintain a balance between cell survival and programmed cell death (apoptosis). Genistein is known to have anti-oxidant property and is a phytoestrogen, which targets estrogen and androgen-mediated signalling pathways in the processes of carcinogenesis. Moreover, genistein is also found to be a potent inhibitor of angiogenesis and metastasis (see Sarkar and Li, 2002 for comprehensive treatment.).

P72. *Green tea* (EGCG as in text) reduces IGF-1 and induces apoptosis. It inhibits Bcl-2, PI3 Kinase, VEGF, UPA. It has been shown that EGCG limits the progression of PC through inhibition of angiogenesis and metastasis, and it is thought to do this by interfering with the IGF-1/IGFBP-3 signalling pathway (Adhami et al.,2004).

EGCG is synergistic with COX-2 inhibitors with resultant slowing of the growth of PC. That is to say, each triggers cellular pathways that, combined, are more powerful than either agent alone. EGCG suppresses androgen receptor signalling and PSA expression in different progression stages of LNCaP prostate cancer cells (Chuu C et al., 2009).

A study carried out by researchers in the Feist-Weiller Cancer Center, LSU Health Sciences Center-Shreveport, USA, found that men with prostate cancer who consumed the active compounds found in green tea had considerable reduction in serum markers predictive of prostate cancer progression. The study has been published in *Cancer Prevention Research*. Reported in Medical News Today, June, 2009.

P72. *Curcumin.* Rather than quote all the references, perhaps it will suffice to list some of the well documented properties of curcumin and leave it for the technically minded reader to search further in Google if desired. Here follows such an abbreviated list:

Curcumin down-regulates transactivation and expression of AR, activator protein-1 (AP-1), nuclear factor NFkB, and CREB (cAMP response element-binding protein)-binding protein (CBP). It is a specific COX-2 (cycloxygenase) inhibitor as well as a LOX inhibitor reducing the synthesis of PGE2, LTB4 and 5-HETE *in vitro* and *in vivo*. See also P80.

P72. *Silymarin.* The silibinin/silymarin extract from St Mary's milk thistle has remarkable positive actions on prostate cancer cells. Singh et al., (2003) showed that it alters cell cycle progression and inhibits mitogenic and cell survival signallinginvolving EGF-1 receptor and NFkB in PC cells. They observed that silymarin inhibits VEGF and inhibits advanced human PC DU145 tumour xenograft growth in nude mice, as well as cell proliferation, apoptosis and angiogenesis.

A most extensive coverage of the subject is to be found in an article by Singh and Agarwal (2006), including a table of numerous actions of this novel compound in relation to prostate cancer.

P72. *Cinnamon* About half a teaspoon of cinnamon twice a day has been found to reduce insulin spikes and increase insulin sensitivity in cells. It appears that a hydroxychalcone derived from cinnamon functions as a mimetic for insulin in adipocytes or fat cells. For more information on the effects of cinnamon on glucose and insulin and the mechanisms of action, see Khan et al., 2003.

P73. *Pomegranate* induces Bax & Bak (pro-apoptotic). Inhibits Bcl-xL & Bcl-2. Induces WAF/p21 & KIP1/p27. Decreases cyclins D1, D2 and E. Decreases cdk2, cdk4, cdk6 expression. Increased average PSADT from 15 months to 54 months in the Pantuck trials. Produces acute inhibition of *in vitro* proliferation of LNCaP, PC3 & DU145 cell lines. These properties are dealt with in detail by Malik A et al., 2005. The reader might also like to study the Memorial Sloan-Kettering Cancer Centre Information site About Herbs/pomegranate. Further actions of the juice which impact on prostate tumour growth are explained, and the site offers an interesting and informative section on oestrogens.

P73. *Quercetin* inhibits phospholipase, blocks LOX & COX. Inhibits TGF-a induced COX-2 action. Inhibits mutant p53. Induces cell cycle arrest. Inhibits tyrosine kinase & Ras. Increases the ratio Bax/Bcl-2. See P74.

P73. *Resveratrol.* The anti-cancer actions of resveratrol are due primarily to cell cycle arrest, upregulation of p53 and Bax, together with down-regulation of survivin, cyclin D, Bcl-2 and IAP. It activates caspases and suppresses various transcription factors. In particular resveratrol inhibits COX-2, 5-LOX, VEGF, IL-6, AR and PSA. These properties and more may be found in an article by Aggarwal et al., 2004.

P73. *Selenium.* As selenite, may normalize the immune system. Reduces transcription of AR, NFkB, PKC. Synergistic with vitamin E. Critical for Quinone Reductase. Enhances caspase-mediated cleavage of PARP and assists in upregulation of p53. See article by Keck and Finley 2004 and their references.

P74. *Serenoa (saw palmetto)* See also P78. It reduces IGF-1 signaling. It is a potent phytoestrogen, inhibits types 1&2 5a-reductase, affects androgen receptor binding with ligand.

P74. *Vitamin C* reduces NF-kB (IL-6). The controversy over the effectiveness of vitamin C in cancer therapy is a continuing one. A balanced commentary is provided by the National Institutes of Health Office of Dietary Supplements web site.

www.dietary-supplements.info.nih.gov/factsheets/vitaminc.asp.

P74. *Vitamin E.* As mentioned in the text, there is a wealth of literature endorsing vitamin E – in the appropriate forms – for prostate cancer. Likewise for selenium – the two often being coupled together as a treatment. Recently a program which had been studying the therapeutic effect of selenium and vitamin E – called the SELECT program – was cancelled. It was decided that the results were so poor that it was not worth while continuing the study. This has led of course to very unfavourable publicity for both selenium and vitamin E.

It should be said, however, that good scientists have questioned the study design. One argument is that the participants in the study were healthy with quite high levels of selenium – whereas it would have been more appropriate to use subjects deficient in the substance to see if using it could have an effect. Secondly, the form of selenium chosen was incorrect – the literature supports the notion that selenium as selenite could be expected to achieve better results than the methionine form used. Similarly with vitamin E – they used dl-tocopherol in the study, whereas recent literature clearly endorses the preferred use of the complete eight forms of vitamin E, rather than the one form taken in the study. There is also a question about the dosage of vitamin E.

The above information on the arguments against the SELECT study design were supplied as a personal communication by Dr Graham Lyons, a senior agronomist and expert in phytonutrients from the University of Adelaide. Professor Sali from the National Institute of Integrative Medicine continues to recommend both vitamin E and selenium in the appropriate forms. I take both products daily.

P77. *Fish oil* has a strong anti-inflammatory action. Chronic inflammation is now thought to be a factor in the development of PC. EPA and DHA selectively inhibit COX-2 without impacting COX-1, and they reduce the synthesis of cytokines TNF-alpha and IL-1. Supplementation with fish oil has a profound effect on the immune system, significantly increasing the T-helper/T-suppressor cell ratio in cancer patients with solid tumours (Cogas et al., 1995).

P72. *Natural Health Products* or NHPs target various molecular pathways besides angiogenesis, including epidermal growth factor receptor (EGFR), the HER-2/neu gene, the cyclooxygenase-2 enzyme, the NF-kB transcription factor, the protein kinases, Bcl-2 protein, and coagulation pathways. The herbalist has access to hundreds of years of observational data on the anticancer activity of many herbs. Laboratory studies are confirming the knowledge that is already documented in traditional texts.

P73. *Serenoa (saw palmetto)* is also an inhibitor of aromatase, 5alpha-reductase (types 1 and 2), COX-2 (cycloxygenase-2) and 5-LOX (5-Lipoxygenase). All of these actions are of great importance in PC. It reduces IGF-1 signalling and interferes with ligand binding to androgen receptor. All the above and more information can be found at the web site www.herbmed.org

P74. *Beta-sitosterol* activates the sphingomyelin cycle to induce apoptosis in LNCaP cells. It also decreases the size and the extent of (breast) tumour metastases in vivo. The sterol also significantly increases Fas levels and caspase-8 activity (Awad et al., 2007).

P78. *Quercetin* The enthusiastic reader may wish to read an excellent paper by Lakhanpal and Rai (2007). The article and references quoted reveal just what an extraordinary phytonutrient this is. Amongst other functions, it inhibits phospholipase, blocks LOX & COX. It inhibits TGF-a induced COX-2 action, inhibits mutant p53. It induces cell cycle arrest and inhibits tyrosine kinase & Ras. Quercetin increases the ratio of Bax/Bcl-2.

P79. *Ginger* or 6-Gingerol (Seong-Ho, 2007). It is a natural product of ginger, has been known to possess anti-tumorigenic and pro-apoptotic activities. However, the mechanisms by which it prevents cancer are not well understood in human colorectal cancer. Cyclin D1 is a proto-oncogene that is overexpressed in many cancers and plays a role in cell proliferation through activation by beta-catenin signalling. Nonsteroidal anti-inflammatory drug (NSAID)-activated gene-1 (NAG-1) is a cytokine associated with pro-apoptotic and anti-tumorigenic properties. In the present study, we examined whether 6-gingerol influences cyclin D1 and NAG-1 expression and determined the mechanisms by which 6-gingerol affects the growth of human colorectal cancer cells in vitro. 6-Gingerol treatment suppressed cell proliferation and induced apoptosis and G(1) cell cycle arrest. Subsequently, 6-gingerol suppressed cyclin D1 expression and induced NAG-1 expression. Cyclin D1 suppression was related to inhibition of beta-catenin translocation and cyclin D1 proteolysis. Furthermore, experiments using inhibitors and siRNA transfection confirm the involvement of the PKCepsilon and glycogen synthase kinase (GSK)-3beta pathways in 6-gingerol-induced NAG-1 expression. The results suggest that 6-gingerol stimulates apoptosis through upregulation of NAG-1 and G(1) cell cycle arrest through down-regulation of cyclin D1. Multiple mechanisms appear to be involved in 6-gingerol action, including protein degradation as well as beta-catenin, PKCepsilon, and GSK-3beta pathways. *[Author's note: Most of the above relates to PC as well.]*

P79. *Panax Ginseng* In the on-line edition of Phytotherapy Research, March 9th 2009, Varja et al., reported the effect of ginseng on the expression of genes BCl2 and Cyclin D. It seems that this is the mechanism by which the herb enhances apoptosis.

P80. *Curcumin* is a specific inhibitor of COX-2, the 'bad cyclo-oxygenase (Goel et al., 2001) and for PC sufferers this may be its most valuable action. It has also been shown that curcumin has a synergistic action with PEITC.

But it does far more than this. The reader who wishes to learn more about this powerful compound and its anti-cancer activity, you will find an outstanding summary on the internet by Guarisanka Sa and Tanya Das (2008).

P86. *Lowering of PSA.* Re The question as to whether lowering of PSA by any therapy might not reflect true impact on the cancer.

After recurrence, a rising PSA level is a strong indicator of the existence of extraprostatic micrometastases – that is, tiny cancers starting up outside the prostate – and the rate of further PSA rise is the best single predictor of survival (Saxe et al., 2005). Those men with a PSA doubling time (PSADT) of less than 10months have a 65% to 75% 5-year risk of developing metastatic disease, whereas those with PSADT greater than 10months have a risk of only 10% to 20% (Saxe et al., 2001).

It is of interest that while Ornish and his team (2008) felt unable to come to definitive conclusions as to the effect their regime was having on the progress of the PC (mainly because of insufficient numbers), they had established compelling indicators. For example, they found that 48 genes were up-regulated and 453 genes were down-regulated.

The Ornish team found also that serum from the intervention participants decreased the growth of LNCaP cells almost eight times more than serum from the control group, suggesting again that comprehensive lifestyle changes may have affected tumour growth as well as PSA. The changes in PSA and in LNCaP growth were also significantly related to the extent to which the participants had changed their lifestyle, and this also supports the hypothesis that such an intervention may affect the progression of PC. Others have performed investigations which support this (Wang et al., 1995; Denmark-Wahnefried et al., 2001; Tymchuk et al., 2001).

Ornish et al., considered the possibility that the decrease in PSA was an 'artifact', They make the compelling observation, that two recent articles failed to show any effect on PSA levels in men who did *not* have PC after four years on a diet quite similar to theirs (Shike et al., 2002; Eastham et al., 2003). For a PSA lowering effect to occur under similar conditions *only* in men who *did* have PC leaves little doubt that the cancer itself is being impacted by the intervention and therefore expressing less of the antigen.

Nicholas Vogelzand and colleagues in their recent *Comprehensive Textbook of Genitourinary Oncology* (2009), review the literature on the subject of androgen ablation and its real rather than 'artifactual' biological effects. They discuss changes in histology or how the cells look under a microscope, tumor size and volume, effects on tumor grading, clinical studies including survival times, and they specifically address the above question with references.

More on the proposed trial relating to the 'artifact' effect, p85.

Investigations/assays such as MRI/CT, colour Doppler, bone scans, testosterone, DHT, PCA3, calcitriol, fasting insulin and oestrone levels, or circulating cancer cells could be monitored. See Nogueira et al., 2009 for discussion of new biomarkers.

Prostatic Acid Phosphatase (PAP) and Chromogranin A levels could be followed for those men with advanced cancer. It might then be possible to detect molecular or other changes which, together with any clinical improvement such as pain relief, would demonstrate that the cancer itself has been impacted for the better. This would negate the idea that the lowering of the PSA was an artifact.

Donald Murphy my urologist, however, makes these further points which are relevant: "PAP is not prostate specific. Reverse trans-scriptase testing and cancer cells in the blood stream have also been investigated but have not proved helpful. PSA lowering is only one part of the story. PSA is in fact a normal substance found in normal males and while it is prostate specific, it is not prostate cancer specific. Elevated levels do not mean cancer."

Further to the discussion about the likely negative actions of PSA, Sutkowski and associates (1999) suggested that PSA may regulate the volume of stromal tissue in men with BPH. PSA cleaves insulin-like growth factor–binding protein-3 (IGFBP3), which decreases its affinity for insulin-like growth factor (IGF-1), which is an epithelial cell mitogen. Dissociation of the IGFBP3 complex makes IGF-1 available to bind to its receptor and to stimulate cell proliferation.

P79. *Reishi mushroom* inhibits constitutively active transcription factors nuclear factor kappa B (NF-kappaB) and AP-1, which results in the inhibition of expression of urokinase-type plasminogen activator (uPA) and its receptor uPAR. Ganoderma lucidum also suppresses cell adhesion and cell migration of highly invasive breast and prostate cancer cells, suggesting its potency to reduce tumor invasiveness. This study by Sliva was reported in Integ. Cancer Ther. 2003;2:358–364.

P79. *Pygeum* inhibits the growth of PC-3 and LNCaP cells and induces apoptosis, It down-regulates ER-alpha. Pygeum inhibited the growth of PC-3 and LNCaP cells and in vivo TRAMP mouse model (Shenouda et al., 2007).

P92. *Exercise* also lowers circulating TNF, CRP and IL-6.

P103&57. *The Ornish trials.* It is significant that a set of *RAS* family oncogenes (*RAN*) was among the genes down-regulated, and of course the *RAS* family are highly expressed in PC.

They also found that *SHOC2* was among the down-regulated genes, and this gene encodes a protein which is essential in MAPK activation by growth factors. *SHOC2* is proposed to be an attractive therapeutic target in the treatment of cancers with up-regulated MAPK activity, of which PC is one.

They found down-regulation of important IGF pathway genes such as *IGF1R, PIK3C2A.*

All this means that they had identified significant modulation of biological processes with critical roles in tumourigenesis after the lifestyle intervention.

P102. *More on Prostasol.* While standard full androgen blockade or deprivation involves intervention in the hypothalamo-pituitary axis to produce chemical castration, Prostasol impinges on the prostate and the tumor directly as well as enhancing the immune system. So it does not involve quite the same initiating pathways as in the case of standard hormonal therapy, nevertheless the physiological effects are the same – dramatic drop in levels of PSA, testosterone, DHT and so on. The mechanisms by which Prostasol achieves this are now fairly well understood as discussed in Chapter 5 on Supplements.

P102. With regard to the on-going maintenance with synthetic Proscar or Avodart, there are two points which could be made. First, some natural herbs such as epilobium inhibit not only 5-alpha-reductase but also aromatase, the enzyme which turns testosterone into estradiol, the 'bad' estrogen for PC sufferers. Second, after androgen ablation, the androgen receptors (AR) in the cancer cells almost invariably develop strategies to survive on virtually no androgen. Dr Leibowitz's approach seems to avoid this, although he has back-up plans if resistance (or more accurately, hypersensitivity to androgen) does emerge. Professor Ben Pfeifer has different tactics in this situation – he adds zeolite and biobran to the Prostasol. Other practitioners of this approach increase the amount of sterols in their mix.

Once DHT is reduced using either Proscar or Avodart, could the cancer cells become aggressive as with conventional androgen blockade? Perhaps since there is now a higher level of ordinary testosterone in the system, this keeps the cancer cells 'happy' enough not to go aggressive. The key question remains, what causes the cancer cells to become independent? Charles Myers has written a comprehensive three-part treatise on this question, though the question remains largely unresolved (Myers, 2003).

Whichever primary approach is chosen, the thrust of this book is that it should be part of a holistic, multi-targeted program incorporating Pro-active Surveillance. Following is a model which our team is currently thinking through, as it relates to my current regime.

a) Continue the Sali/Ornish lifestyle approach while monitoring PC activity (via PSA kinetics and other biomarkers or investigations if and as required).
b) Perhaps add sterols/sterolins to the supplements discussed in Chapter 5. There is a product called Natur-leaf (US) which contains a natural blend of these compounds, the main one being beta-sitosterol and its glycoside.
c) If and when required – that is, if the PC looks like progressing – take Prostasol for 13 months together with a 5-alpha-reductase inhibitor. The same inhibitor would then continue as on-going maintenance to emulate the successful Leibowitz protocol.
d) If and when required – that is, if ever androgen independence occurred – follow either the Pfeifer regime with zeolite and biobran, or the Leibowitz protocol and, if necessary, his 'anti-angiogenic cocktail'. This consists of a *very* mild regime of chemotherapy, but taken in such a way as not to disrupt the patients' ability to enjoy an excellent quality of life.

Dr Leibowitz argues that, "Prostate cancer is exceptionally and almost universally responsive to treatment. While metastatic prostate cancer cannot be cured, it is highly treatable and controllable. The goal of treating patients with metastatic cancer is to turn their illness into a chronic disease, much like hypertension or diabetes. You don't cure those diseases, you successfully treat and control them. It is not necessary to cure most patients with metastatic prostate cancer in order for them to live a normal

> lifespan. Our goal is to make prostate cancer cells 'hibernate'; to make them *dormant*. Remember that 80% of men in their 80's have prostate cancer. Most of us live with prostate cancer and die *with* it, not *from* it. Our realistic, achievable goal is to control metastatic prostate cancer. For almost all of the patients treated at Compassionate Oncology Medical Group, this goal continues to be successfully accomplished."

A further element to be considered in each individual case, is the advisability or otherwise of early de-bulking as mentioned above. From my point of view, Irreversible Electroporation (IRE) or Photo Dynamic Therapy (PDT) would be the ways of choice. Both have been discussed in Chapter 7. Unfortunately at this time, IRE has been used only on a few men with PC in the USA (though with very successful results). PDT, though quite promising, has not yet been formally proven to work in prostate cancer. Professor Sali and research staff at the National Institute of Integrative Medicine hope, in the near future, to do such trials using this 'minimalist' intervention.

Glossary of Terms

(On-line medical dictionaries are useful too)

Androgen deprivation therapy: In prostate cancer, treatment with drugs that minimise the effect of testosterone in the body so as to slow or stop the growth of the cancer. Also called androgen ablation. There are two common approaches to the therapy, intermittent and continuous. For further details, the reader may wish to search Google for names like Nicholas Bronowski, Charles Myers, Robert Leibowitz.

Angiogenesis: The formation of new blood vessels. Angiogenesis enables tumours to develop their own blood supply which helps them to survive and grow.

Androgens: Male sex hormones. The most active male hormone, testosterone, is produced by the testes. Other male hormones are produced by the adrenal glands.

Anti-oxidant: A nutrient that inhibits oxidation and therefore the deterioration of cells through the action of oxygen or peroxides, and especially through the action of free radicals (very reactive oxygen species).

Arachidonic acid: an omega-6 fatty acid which stimulates the progression of PC, but only after its conversion to one of several powerful hormones (see eicosanoids below).

Bcl-2: Stands for B-cell lymphoma 2. In fact there are many members of this family of genes and the proteins they generate. Some encourage apoptosis (for example Bax) whereas some are anti-apoptotic (for example Bcl-2 itself).

Benign prostate hyperplasia or enlargement (BPH): Non-cancerous enlargement of the prostate due to excessive growth of normal prostate tissue.

Bioflavanoid: The colouring pigment in fruit and vegetables. Many can prevent cell damage due to free radicals, unstable molecules which may be produced by oxidation.

Biopsy: Removal of tissue for diagnosis. The sample is then examined under the microscope to see if cancerous cells are present.

BMI: Body/Mass Index, the ratio of one's weight in kg divided by the square of the height in metres. Should be in the low twenties.

Brachytherapy: Radio therapy given from within the prostate by inserting radioactive 'seeds' directly into the gland.

Cancer: Refers to the various types of malignant growths or tumours that contain cells growing uncontrolled and invading adjacent tissues. They may metastasize to distant tissues.

Cells: The 'building blocks' of the body which are adapted for different functions. Normal cells can divide and reproduce themselves exactly.

CGA: Chromogranin A, a chemical (peptide) found in the blood of men with advanced PC.

Clinically evident: Evident by direct observation or examination.

COX: Cycloxygenase, an enzyme which, in the context of PC, acts on arachidonic acid to produce prostaglandins.

Cross-talk: molecules which act in cell-signalling may 'cross boundaries' and interact with other pathways as well, thus producing multiple responses.

Cryosurgery: Uses freezing to kill cells (in the cancerous prostate for example).

DHT or (5 alpha-dihydrotestosterone): a male hormone which is converted from testosterone within the prostate by an enzyme called 5-alpha reductase. It is much more potent than testosterone.

Disease-specific survival: The percentage of people who have survived a particular disease such as PC after a given treatment after a specific time interval.

DHEA: Dehydroepiandrosterone (DHEA) is a steroid produced by the adrenal glands. It may be transformed into testosterone, estrogen or other steroids. It exists as either DHEA or in the sulfated form known as DHEA-S.

'Differentiation': Refers to the difference between normal cells as they appear under a microscope, and cancerous cells which look abnormal, perhaps with a large, deformed nucleus and so on.

Digital rectal examination (DRE): an examination of the prostate through the wall of the rectum. The doctor inserts a finger into the rectum and feels the shape of the gland so as to detect any irregularities such as cancer.

Doubling time: The time taken for the PSA level to double, for example from 2ng/ml to 4ng/ml and it is thus a reliable measure of how fast the cancer is growing.

EGF-R: Epidermal Growth Factor Receptor.

Eicosanoids: are substances made by enzymes from arachidonic acid. There are four families of these compounds which derive either from omega-3 or omega-6 fatty acids. Prostaglandins are one such family. A particular compound derived from arachidonic acid is 5-HETE or 5-hydroxyeicosatetraenoic acid which has been shown to strongly promote cancer cancer growth. The eicosanoids are signalling molecules (both intra- and extra-cellular) and they exert control over many systems such as those involved with inflammation and immunity.

Endo-rectal: Within the rectum, as in an MRI probe focusing on the prostate through the rectal wall.

Enzymes: Protein catalysts produced by cells that are critical in chemical reactions and in synthesizing most compounds in the body. Each enzyme performs a specific function.

Epidermis: Outer layer of the skin.

Epidemiology: The study of causes, distribution, and control of disease in given populations.

Epigenetic: Refers to changes not directly affecting chromosomal DNA sequence, but which nevertheless can affect gene expression (phenotype).

Epilobium: a natural herb which has 5-alpha reductase and aromatase inhibitory activity. It has a long history of usefulness in prostate disorders and scientific underpinning is emerging to explain its mechanisms of action. It contains a high level of beta-sitosterol.

Epithelial: Related to epithelium, the covering of external and internal surfaces of the body such as the lining of blood vessels or the lining of the oesophagus.

ER-alpha: Estrogen Receptor-alpha. In terms of PC, ER-alpha is not favourable whereas ER-beta is favourable.

External beam radiotherapy (EBRT): Radiotherapy given from a source outside the body.

Extracellular Matrix or ECM: The extracellular tissue which provides support to the cells. It has other functions and its penetration is involved in the invasive stage and spread of PC.

Fatty Acids: Chemical chains of carbon, hydrogen, and oxygen atoms that are part of lipids (fats) and triglycerides. Cholesterol is one example, as are EPA (eicosapentanoic acid) and DHA (docosahexaenoic acid).

Five-year survival rate: A scientific measure used to determine the success of a treatment. It measures the number of people who are alive five years after a certain treatment.

Free to total PSA ratio: The PSA in the bloodstream can bind to a protein. This is called 'bound' PSA. In men with BPH, there tends to be more 'free' or 'unbound' PSA than in men with PC. This test compares the ratio of unbound PSA to total PSA.

Gene: A segment of DNA which directs the production of an enzyme, which itself will be involved in the passing on of hereditary characteristics. So genes are factors which determine the growth and behaviour of cells. They are inherited from both parents and so there are two genes for each characteristic (except in sex cells since the chromosomes are unpaired).

Genotype and phenotype: Genotype refers to the genetic composition of our cells; phenotype refers to the way the genotype is actually expressed, or how we look.

GI: The glycaemic index (GI) is a ranking of foods on a scale from 0 to 100 according to the extent to which they raise blood sugar levels. High GI foods result in higher and more rapid increases in blood glucose levels.

Gleason score: A way of grading cancer cells. A pathologist identifies the two most common tissue patterns and grades them from 1 (least aggressive) to 5 (most aggressive). The Gleason score consists of two numbers which represent the most common and the next most common types of cells to give a score out of ten (for example, 3+4=7).

Grade Shift: Prostate cancer, on repeat biopsy study may have an alteration in the Gleason score.

Gynecomastia: Breast enlargement.

Hormones: Chemical substances secreted by organs in the body which are carried by the bloodstream and usually influence cells some distance from the source of production. Hormones signal particular enzymes to act and thus regulate such functions as blood sugar and insulin levels. Examples would be testosterone, oestrogens and melatonin.

Hormone resistance: Even after primary therapy, prostate cancer cells may develop which can survive and grow without male hormones. The cancer is then said to be resistant.

Hyperinsulinaemia: Excess of insulin in the blood.

Insulin resistance: The action of insulin is no longer as effective as it should be, leading to hyperinsulinaemia.

Integrative medicine: Medicine which takes a 'holistic' approach to health and disease, incorporating mind-body interaction, nutrition and lifestyle in general as fundamental factors in well-being.

Interleukin-6: A cellular product which increases secretion of antibodies by B lymphocytes. Over-expression of IL-6 contributes to prostate cancer progression.

Isoform: Proteins which can exist in different versions, being very similar in structure. They may be generated by the same gene or by different genes.

Localised prostate cancer: Prostate cancer which has not spread beyond the prostate gland.

Locally advanced prostate cancer: Cancer which has spread beyond the prostate capsule itself but is still confined to the prostate and immediate region.

LOX: Lipoxygenase, an enzyme which acts on the omega-6 fatty acid, arachidonic acid to produce compounds which are harmful in PC.

Lymph nodes: Lymph glands found all over the body but easier to feel under the jaw, in the armpits and groin. They 'filter' foreign substances and usually become inflamed and swollen if there is an infection nearby. The filtering action may also trap cancer cells from other parts of the body.

Magnetic resonance imaging (MRI): A method of imaging the inside of the body using magnetic forces and without using X-rays.

Malignant: Cancerous.

McNeal model: J.E. McNeal was a pioneer in prostate cancer anatomy who first described the three zones (central, transitional and peripheral) of prostate architecture. He once remarked that, the prostate, both malignant and normal, had "a tremendous variety of architectural forms, in contrast to other organs which are rather dull, with everything looking the same."

Median: Middle score of many in a survey or study.

Medical oncologist: A cancer specialist who uses chemotherapy.

Melatonin: Hormone produced by the pineal gland which controls sleep-wake cycles. Melatonin may be used in treating PC.

Meta-analysis: Statistically combining the results of several studies of the same problem.

Metabolic syndrome: A condition also called insulin-resistance syndrome. Sufferers are usually obese, have high blood pressure and insulin resistance and are at high risk of cardiovascular disease and diabetes.

Metabolite: A product of metabolism.

Metastasis/metastasise: The spread of cancer away from the site of origin.

Mitogenic: Stimulates mitosis, as in stimulating cancer growth.

Mitosis: Cell division which produces 'daughter cells' identical with the original cell.

Naturopath: One who uses natural herbs and procedures in the treatment of disease.

Neoplastic: Tissue growing abnormally and more rapidly than normal. May be cancerous.

'Number needed to treat': Here is an example from prostate surgery; between 80 and 90 prostatectomies would need to be performed for each PC death (which would be) avoided in a 'favourable risk, screen-detected population'.

Oncologist: A specialist in the treatment of cancer (see medical oncologist and radiation oncologist).

PAP: Prostatic acid phosphatase, an enzyme which is increased in progressing PC, especially metastasising PC.

Pathogenic: causing disease.

Pathologist: A doctor who specialises in the examination of cells and tissue removed from the body.

PC-3: A PC cell type which is the 'classic' cell line of the disease, and which has strong metastatic potential.

Phase 11 enzymes: Carcinogen defence enzymes in the liver.

'Phyto-therapy': Therapy using plant products.

PI3-kinase: Phosphoinositide 3-kinase, member of a biochemical cascade or pathway which has a bad effect on PC. It is involved with insulin (to regulate glucose uptake) and a tumour suppressor gene called PTEN.

Polyphenols: Chemical compounds containing more than one phenol unit per molecule. A phenol is an alcohol.

Prostate: The gland in men which surrounds the neck of the bladder and the urethra and produces a fluid that forms part of semen.

Prostatectomy: Removal of the prostate gland.

Prostate specific antigen (PSA): A protein produced by prostate cells. It is usually found in the blood in larger than normal amounts if prostate cancer is present.

Used as a test for prostate cancer or to monitor its recurrence.

Protease: Enzyme which breaks up proteins.

PSA velocity: A measure of how quickly the PSA rises.

Radiation: Energy in the form of waves such X-rays.

Randomised controlled study: A trial in which subjects are randomly chosen either to receive a treatment or intervention, or to receive a placebo (such as a 'sugar pill'). The latter group are called the 'controls', and the aim is to see whether the intervention produces a result which the control group does not experience.

Receptor: a protein molecule on the cell surface or inside the cell which binds to a 'ligand' or specific compound such as a hormone.

Refractory: Resistant to treatment.

5-alpha Reductase: Enzyme which changes testosterone to DHT.

Stage/staging: The process of determining the extent of the disease. A system of describing how far the cancer has spread.

Sympathetic and parasympathetic: Two branches of the (peripheral) nervous system: sympathetic refers to the 'fight-and-flight' (adrenalin) response to a stimulus, while parasympathetic refers to the 'house-keeping' or relaxation response – the 'normal' mode of the nervous system.

Synergism: refers to the way various compounds can work together, so that the combined effect is greater than the effect from either substance alone. A multi-pronged approach to PC has been mentioned earlier. The attack needs to address all of the six/seven processes, hormonal balance, cell signalling, cell cycle regulation and differentiation, cell survival/apoptosis, neo-angiogenesis and carcinogen metabolism Hence the best nutrients will be those which will cover as many of these processes as possible and the more synergism the better.

Below are some well established combinations of natural compounds which exhibit synergism:

- Quercetin, ellagic acid and resveratrol
- Quercetin and silibinin
- Quercetin and EGCG (Green tea extract)
- EGCG and vitamin D
- Curcumin and CoQ10
- Curcumin and EGCG
- Curcumin and PEITC
- Vitamin E and lycopene
- Vitamin E and vitamin C, beta-carotene, selenium and zinc

Testosterone: The main sex hormone that induces and maintains the changes that take place in males at puberty.

T1/T2 grading of PC: The TNM system of PC grading refers to **T**umour stage, lymph **N**ode stage and **M**etastasis stage. So T1 is the first stage of PC and means that digital examination did not present any lumps indicative of cancer. Also no lymph node involvement and no metastases were observed. T2 and T3 would be next stages of progression. For example, T2 means palpable during rectal examination but confined to prostate, and so on. Each T stage is also divided into three levels, a, b and c. These refer to how the definitive cancer was discovered. For example, the c in T1c means that the cancer was discovered after biopsy.

TNF-alpha: Tumour Necrosis Factor-alpha. A cell product involved in inflammation by regulating immune cells. It can induce apoptosis and inhibit the growth of tumours, but if disregulated or if overexpressed, it can stimulate cancer.

TNM system: A system for staging cancer, depending on the size and invasiveness of the tumour, whether lymph nodes are affected, and whether there is metastasis.

Tumorigenesis: Causing cancer.

uPA: Urokinase Plasminogen Activator.

Urethra: The tube which carries urine and ejaculate along the length of the penis and to the outside of the body.

Urologist: Surgeons who specialise in treating urogenital tract diseases.

VEGF: Vascular Endothelial Growth Factor. Assists angiogenesis so not helpful for PC.

Vitamin D: A fat-soluble vitamin essential to one's health. Regulates the amount of calcium and phosphorus in the blood by improving their absorption and utilization.

Necessary for normal growth and formation of bones and teeth. For Vitamin D only, 1mcg translates to 40 IU.

Well-differentiated tumours: Look like normal cells under the microscope.

Xenograft: Graft of tissue, for example a tumour, from an animal of one species to an animal of another species. Commonly human PC tissue to mice.

References

Ades T. PC-SPES: Current Evidence and Remaining Questions. Cancer J Clin, 2001;51: 100.

Adhami V et al., Oral consumption of Green Tea Polyphenols Inhibits IGF-1 signalling in an autochthonous Mouse Model of Prostate Cancer. Cancer Research, 2004;64: 8715-8722.

Aggarwal, B et al., Role of resveratrol in prevention and therapy of cancer: Preclinical and clinical studies. Anticancer Res. 2004;24: 3-60.

Allen N et al., Animal products, protein, calcium and prostate cancer risk: the Prospective European Investigation into Cancer and Nutrition. Br J Cancer, 2008;98: 1574-1581.

Antoni MH et al., The influence of bio-behavioural factors on tumour biology: Pathways and mechanisms. *Nature Reviews Cancer* 2006; 6(3): 240-248.

Astin J et al., Mind-body medicine: state of the science, implications for practice. J Amer. Board Fam. Practice, 2003;16; 131-147.

Awad A et al., Beta-sitosterol activates Fas signalling in human breast cancer cells. Phytomed. 2007;14: 747-754.

Barnard R et al., Prostate cancer: another aspect of the insulin-resistance syndrome? Blackwell Synergy – Obesity Reviews, 2002;3: 303-308.

Barocas D. Active surveillance underutilized in prostate cancer. Updated follow-up of active surveillance with selected delayed intervention for localized prostate cancer, Multidisciplinary Prostate Cancer Symposium in Orlando, Florida, 2006.

Ben-Eliyahu S. Stress, NK cells and cancer: Still a promissory note. Brain, Behaviour and Immunity, 2007;21: 881-887.

Ben-Eliyahu S et al., Suppression of NK cell and of resistance to metastasis by stress: A role for catecholamines and beta-adrenoceptors. Neuroimmunomodulation, 2000;8: 154-164.

Ben Sahra I et al., The anti-diabetic drug Metformin exerts an anti-tumoral effect *in vitro* and *in vivo* through a decrease in Cyclin D1 level. Oncogene, 2008;27: 3576-3586.

Carlson L and Garland S. Effect of Psychsocial Intervention on Psychneuroendocrine Outcomes in Cancer Patients: Where Do We Go From Here? In 'Psychoneurology Research Trends'. Ed. Martina Czerbska. Nova Scotia Publishers 2007;213-257.

Choi S et al., D,L-sulforaphane-induced cell death in human prostate cancer cells is regulated by inhibitor of apoptosis family proteins and Apaf-1. Carcinogen. 2007;28: 151-162.

Choo R et al., Feasibility study: watchful waiting for localized low to intermediate grade prostate carcinoma with selective delayed intervention based on PSA, histological and/or clinical progression. J Urol. 2002;167: 1664-1669.

Chuu C et al., Suppression of androgen receptor signalling and PSA expression by EGCG in different progression stages of LNCaP prostate cancer cells. Cancer Lett. 2009;275: 86-92.

Clark A and Lelkes O. 'Deliver us from evil': religion as insurance. Papers on Economics of Religion, Dept of Economic Theory and Economic History, University of Granada, 2006. Paper No. 06/03.

Cogas C et al., The effect of omega-3 polyunsaturated fatty acid on T-lymphocyte subsets of patients with solid tumours. Cancer Detect. Prev. 1005;19: 415-417.

Coker KH. Meditation and prostate cancer: integrating a mind/body intervention with traditional therapies. Semin Urol Oncol. 1999;17: 111-118.

Dall'Era MA et al., Active surveillance for early-stage prostate cancer: review of the current literature. Cancer, 2008;112: 1650-1659.

Dall'Era MA & Konety BR. Active surveillance for low-risk prostate cancer: selection of patients and predictors of progression. Nat Clin Pract Urol. 2008;5: 277-283.

Darzynkiewicz Z. Chinese herbal mixture PC SPES in treatment of prostate cancer (review). Int J Oncol. 2000;17: 729-736.

Etzioni R et al., Overdiagnosis due to PSA screening: lessons from US prostate cancer incidence trends. J Natl Cancer Inst.2002;94:981-990.

Ewer T. An integrative Approach. Presented at JAIMA Conference, Australia, September 2008, No 18.

Fahey J et al., Broccoli sprouts: an exceptionally rich source of inducers of enzymes that protect against chemical carcinogens. Proc. Natl. Acad. Sci. 1997;94:10367-10372.

Gaynor Integrative Oncology. Isoflavones and the prevention of prostate disease: is there a role? In Cleveland Clinic Journal of Medicine, Vol 70 No 3: March, 2003.

Giles L et al., Effect of social networks on 10 year survival in very old Australians: the Australian longitudinal study of aging. J. Epidemiol. and Comm. Health, 2005;59: 574-579.

Giovanucci E. Dairy products and risk for aggressive prostate cancer. Cancer Project Symposium, Bethesda, 2006.

Giton F et al., Estrone sulfate (E1S), a prognosis marker for tumor aggressiveness in prostate cancer (PCa). J Steroid Biochem Mol Biol. 2008;109: 158-167.

Goel A et al., Specific inhibition of cyclooxygenase-2 (COX-2) expression by dietary curcumin in HT-29 human colon cancer cells. Cancer Lett. 2001;172: 111-118.

Goodwin J et al., Cause of death in older men after the diagnosis of prostate cancer. J Amer Geriat Soc, 2009;57: 24-30

Goodwin P. Insulin in the adjuvant breast cancer setting: a novel therapeutic target for lifestyle and pharmacologic interventions? J Clin Oncol. 2008;26: 833-834.

Grant W. How strong is the evidence that solar UVB and vitamin D reduce the risk of cancer? Dermato-Endocrinol. 2009;1: 17-24.

Hammarsten J and Hogstedt B. Hyperinsulinaemia: a prospective risk factor for lethal prostate cancer. Eur J Cancer, 2005;41: 2887-2895.

Hollick M. Vitamin D deficiency. A Review. N Engl J. Med. 2007;357: 266-281.

Holz R et al., Beta-sitosterol activates the sphingomyelin cycle and induces apoptosis in LNCaP human prostate cancer cells. Nutr. Cancer, 1998;32: 8-12.

Hsing A et al., Prostate cancer risk and serum levels of insulin and leptin: a population-based study. JNCI, 2001;93: 783-789.

Ingraham B et al., Molecular basis of the potential of vitamin D to prevent cancer. Curr Med Res Opin 2008;24: 139-49.

Johns Hopkins Medicine Health Alerts. Bulletin Nov 7th 2008. Experts now estimate that up to 90% of cancers of the prostate may have a dietary link. New evidence that the progression of prostate cancer may actually be slowed by dietary changes.

Khan A et al., Cinnamon improves glucose and lipids of people with Type 2 diabetes. Diabetes Care, 2003;26: 3215-3218.

Khan M et al., Vitamin D for the management of prostate cancer. Rev Urol. 2004;6: 95-97.

Keck A and Finley J. Cruciferous vegetables: Cancer protective mechanisms of glucosinolate hydrolysis products and selenium. Integr. Cancer Ther. 2004;3: 5-12.

Khan N et al., Apoptosis by dietary factors: the suicide solution for delating cancer growth. Carcinogensis, 2007;28: 233-239.

Kiecolt-Glaser J et al., Psycho-oncology and cancer: psychoneuroimmunology and cancer. 2002 Bulletin European Society for Medical Oncology.

Klotz L. Active surveillance for prostate cancer: For whom? J Clin Oncology, 2005; 23: 8165-8169.

Klotz L. Active surveillance with selective delayed intervention is the way to manage 'good risk' prostate cancer. Nat Clin Pract Urol. 2005;2: 136-142.

Klotz L. (a) What is the best approach for screen-detected low volume cancers? – The case for observation. Urol Oncol. 2008;26: 495-499.

Klotz L. (b) Active surveillance for prostate cancer: trials and tribulations. World J Urol. 2008;26: 437-442.

Krishnan AV et al., Novel pathways that contribute to the anti-proliferative and chemopreventive activities of calcitriol in prostate cancer. J Steroid Biochem Mol Biol. 2007.

Krishnan AV et al.. Inhibition of prostate cancer growth by vitamin D: Regulation of target gene expression. J Cell Biochem 2003; 88: 363-71.

La Cava A. Unravelling the multiple roles of leptin in inflammation and autoimmunity. J Mol Med. 2003.

Lakhanpal P and Rai D. Quercetin: A versatile flavonoid. Internet J. Med. Update. 2007;2: 20-35.

Law JH et al., Phosphorylated Insulin-Like Growth Factor-I/Insulin Receptor Is Present in All Breast Cancer Subtypes and Is Related to Poor Survival. Cancer Res. 2008;68(24):10238–46.

Ledesma N. Nutrition and Prostate cancer. Cancer Supportive Programs National and International, 2005; p1ff.

Lee Seong-Ho et al., Multiple mechanisms are involved in 6-gingerol-induced cell growth arrest and apoptosis in human colorectal cancer cells. Molec. Carcinogen. 2008;47(3):197-208.

Leibovici D et al., Management of prostate cancer with indolent biological potential: from watchful waiting to active surveillance (in Hebrew). Harefuah, 2006;145: 781-780.

Leibowitz, R. Antiangiogenic Cocktail (AAC) (8/2008), formerly 'Leukine (GM-CSF) and Revlimid, the Second

Generation Thalidomide Product' (updated 2/4/2008; originally written 09/2006). Taken from the website www.compassionateoncology.org

Li H et al., A prospective study of plasma selenium levels and prostate cancer risk. J Nat Cancer Inst. 2004:96; 696-703.

Lipton B. The Biology of Belief: Unleashing the power of consciousness, matter and miracles. 2005, Mountain of Love Productions.

Loblaw DA et al., Comparing PSA triggers for treatment for men with prostate cancer on active surveillance. Updated follow-up of active surveillance with selected delayed intervention for localized prostate cancer, Multidisciplinary Prostate Cancer Symposium in Orlando, Florida, 2007.

Lu-Yao M et al., Disease trajectory of untreated localized prostate cancer in elderly men: a population-based study. American Society of Clinical Oncology. Genitourinary Cancers Symposium 2008. Abstract No 10.

Lyons, G et al. Biofortification in the Food Chain and Uses of Selenium and Phytocompounds in Risk Reduction and Control of Prostate Cancer. In 'Development and Uses of Biofortified Agricultural Products.' (Ed. Banuelos G.S and Lin-Qing.) pp 17-44. CRC Press 2009.

Malik A et al., Pomegranate fruit juice for chemoprevention and chemotherapy of prostate cancer. Proc. Nat. Acad. Sci. 2005;102: 14813-14818.

Miller DC et al., Incidence of initial local therapy among men with lower-risk prostate cancer in the US. J Nat Cancer Inst. 2006;98: 1134-1148.

Matilainen, M et al., Regulation of multiple insulin-like growth factor binding protein genes by 1,25-dihydroxyvitaminD3. Nucleic Acids Res. 2005;33: 5521-5532.

McCullough ME et al., Religious involvement and mortality: a meta-analytical review. Health Psych. 2000;19: 211-222.

McLaren DB, McKenzie M, Duncan G, Pickles T. Watchful waiting or watchful progression? Prostate specific antigen doubling times and clinical behavior in patients with early untreated prostate carcinoma. *Cancer.* 1998;82: 342.

Meares, A. A form of intensive meditation associated with the regression of cancer. American Journal of Clinical Hypnosis, 1982 ;25: 114-121.

Meng Q et al., Inhibitory effects of indole-3-carbinol on invasion and migration in human breast cancer cells. Breast Cancer Res Treat. 2000;63: 147-152.

Mohammad M R et al., Down-regulation of Androgen receptor by 3,3-diindolylmethane contributes to inhibition of cell proliferation and induction of apoptosis in both hormone-sensitive LNCaP and insensitive C4-2B prostate cancer cells. Cancer Res, 2007;67: 3310-3319.

Myers C and Myers S. Eating your way to better health: the Prostate Forum Nutrition Guide. Rivanna Health Publications LLC, 2000.

Myers C. Diet and Health. Lecture sponsored by Prostate Cancer Foundation of Australia, Sydney 2000.

Myers C. Androgen resistance (3 parts). Prostate Cancer Research Institute 'Insights', May, 2003 v 6.2.

Myers C. (a) Beating Prostate Cancer: Hormonal Therapy and Diet. Rivanna Health Publications LLC, 2007; p130.

Myers C. (b) Doing nothing until metastatic prostate cancer develops. The Prostate Forum, 2007; Bulletin Vol. 9.9.

Nandeesha H. Insulin: A novel agent in the pathogenesis of prostate cancer. Int Urol Nephrol. 2008 Jul 30. (Epub ahead of print)

Nakamura et al., Curcumin down-regulates AR gene expression and activation in prostate cancer cell lines. Internat. J. Oncology. 2002;21: 825-830.

Nogueira L et al., Other biomarkers for detecting prostate cancer. BJU Int. 2009 Nov. 20th. E-pub ahead of print. PubMed Abstract PMID:19930175.

Olm E et al., Extracellular thiol-dependant selenium uptake dependant on the Xc cystine transporter explains the cancer-specific cytotoxicity of selenite. Proc Nat Acad Sci USA. 2009;106: 11400-11405.

Ornish D et al., Intensive lifestyle changes may affect the progression of prostate cancer. J Urol, 2005;174: 1065-1070.

Ornish D et al., Changes in prostate gene expression in men undergoing an intensive nutrition and lifestyle intervention. Proc Nat Academy Science, 2008;105:8369-8374.

Pantuck AJ et al., Phase 11 Study of pomegranate juice for men with rising prostate-specific antigen following surgery or radiation for prostate cancer. Clin Cancer Res, 2006;12: 4018-4026.

Pantuck AJ et al., Long term follow up of phase 2 study of pomegranate juice for men with prostate cancer shows durable prolongation of PSA doubling time. J Urol, suppl. 2009: 181, 4, abstract 826.

Parker C et al., Repeat biopsy in untreated, clinically localized prostate cancer. American Society of Oncology. 2006 Prostate Cancer Symposium; Abstract No. 34.

Pinsky J. Can natural dietary supplements really impact prostate cancer? Prostate Cancer Research Institute *Insights*, 2007;10: No 1.

Pollack M. Obesity, insulin levels impact prostate cancer survival. In Prostate Cancer Foundation News, 5th October, 2008.

Reiche EM et al., Stress, depression, the immune system, and cancer. *The Lancet Oncology* 2004;5: 617-625.

Sa, G and Ras, T. Anti-cancer effects of curcumin: cycle of life and death. Cell Division;3: 14.

Sali A. Nutrition for healing, prevention and wellness. In Cohen M (Ed). Holistic Healthcare Perspectives, Crows Nest, NSW. Optimal Health Communications, 2006:183-195.

Sali A. Nutrition for health. MJA, 2007;186: 214-216.

Sali A and Vitetta L. Management of Prostate cancer: An integrative approach may reduce the incidence of the disease and slow its progression. Australian Doctor, 24 September, 2007.

Sarkar F and Li Y. Mechanisms of action of cancer chemoprevention by soy isoflavone genistein. Cancer and Metastasis Rev. 2002;21: 265-280.

Saxe G et al., Potential attenuation of disease progression in recurrent prostate cancer with plant-based diet and stress reduction. Integ Cancer Ther. 2006;5: 206-213.

Scholz, M. Can diet really control prostate cancer? Prostate Cancer Research Institute 'Insights', Feb. 2006 vol. 9.

Schussler G et al., The influence of psychosocial factors on the immune system (psychoneuroimmunology) and their role for the incidence and progression of cancer. Psychsom. Med. Psychother. 2001:47; 6-41.

Schwartz G. Vitamin D and intervention trials in prostate cancer: from theory to therapy. Ann Epidemiol. 2008 [Epub ahead of print].

Shenouda N et al., Phytosterol *Pygeum Africanum* regulates prostate cancer *in vitro* and *in vivo*. Endocrine, 2007;31: 72-81.

Shirai, T., Imaida, K., & Ito, N. (2000). Prostate. In: M. Nagao and T. Sugimura (Eds.), Food Born Carcinogenesis. *Current Toxicology Series*, (pp. 270-274). Wiley, Chichester.

Singh R et al., Suppression of advanced human prostate tumour growth in athymic mice by silibinin feeding is associated with decreased cell proliferation, increased apoptosis and inhibited angiogenesis. Cancer Epidemiol. Biomarkers and Prevention, 2003; 12: 933.

Singh RP. *In vivo* suppression of hormone resistant prostate cancer growth by inositol hexaphosphate. Clin Cancer Res. 2004.

Singh R and Agarwal, R. Mechanism of action of novel agents for prostate cancer chemoprevention. Endocrine-related Cancer, 2006;13: 751-778.

Singh P et al., A potential paradox in PC progression: estrogen as the initiating driver. Eur J Cancer, 2008;44: 928-936.

Spiegel D et al., Effect of psychosocial therapy on survival of patients with metastatic breast cancer. Lancet, 1989;2;

888-891.

Swanson G et al., Metastatic prostate cancer: Does treatment of the primary tumour matter? J. Urol. 2006;176: 1292-1298.

Tareen B et al., A 12 Week, Open Label, Phase I/IIa Study Using Apatone® for the Treatment of Prostate Cancer Patients Who Have Failed Standard Therapy. *Int J Med Sci* 2008;5: 62-67.

Taylor P et al., Science peels the onion of selenium effects on prostate carcinogenesis. J Nat. Cancer Inst. 2004:96; 645-647.

Thangapazham R et al., Multiple biological activities of curcumin: a short review. Life Sciences, 2006;208: 2081-2087.

Tucker S, Roundy J, Leibowitz R. Primary Triple Androgen Blockade (TAB) Followed by Finasteride Maintenance (FM) for Clinically Localized Prostate Cancer (CL-CP): Long Term Follow-up and Quality of Life (QOL). 2005 ASCO Prostate Cancer Symposium. See also www.compassionateoncology.org

Van As NJ et al., Active surveillance of low risk localized prostate cancer: baseline predictors of disease progression. American Society of Oncology. 2007 Prostate Cancer Symposium; Abstract No. 319.

Venkateswaren V et al., Association of diet-induced hyperinsulinaemia with accelerated growth of prostate cancer (LNCaP) in xenografts. JNCI, 2007;99: 1793-1800.

Vijayababu M et al., Effects of quercetin on insulin-like growth factors (IGFs) and their binding protein-3 (IGFBP-3) and induction of apoptosis in human prostate cancer cell lines. J carcinog. 2006;5: 10.

Vitetta et al., Mind-body medicine: Stress and its impact on overall health and longevity. Ann. NY Acad. Sci. 2005:1057; 492-505.

Vitetta L & Sali A. Positive thinking, diet, meditation and psychosocial support and its effects on the psychological and physical wellbeing of cancer patients. In: *Third International Congress on Complementary Medicine Research 2008*, Sydney, Australia, (S90-S90). 29-31 March 2008.

Vogelzand N et al. Comprehensive Textbook of Genitourinary Oncolog7. Lippincott, Williams and Wilkins, 2009, pp259-

Wahlqvist M. The truth about soy. The ABC(Australia) Health Report, 12 July 2004.

Wallace JM. Nutritional and botanical modulation of the inflammatory cascade – eicosanoids, cyclooxygenases and lipoxygenases – as an adjunct in cancer therapy. Integ Cancer Ther. 2002;1: 7-37.

Wang J. Genistein chemoprevention of prostate cancer in TRAMP mice. J carcinog. 2007;6: 3.

Wei JT. (University of Michigan in Ann Arbor). Approximately one half of men diagnosed with low-risk prostate cancer undergo surgery or radiation therapy when watchful waiting (Active Surveillance) may have been a more appropriate initial response. The Prostate Cancer Charity, 2007.

Wilkinson G. The effects of diet, aging and disease-states on presystemic elimination and oral drug bioavailability in humans. *Advance Drug Delivery Reviews,* 1997; 27: 129-159.

Wilt T J et al., Systematic review: Comparative effectiveness and harms of treatments for clinically localized prostate cancer. Ann Intern Med. 2008;148: 435-448.

Wright M et al., Supplemental and Dietary Vitamin E Intakes and Risk of Prostate Cancer in a Large Prospective Study. *Cancer Epidemiol Biomarkers & Prevention, 2007;*16: 1128.

Yamanaka-Okumara H. Natto and viscous vegetables in a Japanese style meal suppress postprandial glucose and insulin responses. Asia Pac.J Clin Nutr. 2008;17(4): 663-668.

Yance R and Sagar M. Targeting Angiogenesis With Integrative Cancer Therapies. Integr Cancer Ther. 2006;5: 9-29

Yap, Y et al., γ-Tocotrienol suppresses prostate cancer cell proliferation and invasion through multiple-signalling pathways. Brit. J. Cancer, 2008, 99: 1832–1841.

Young Hong M et al., Pomegranate products and their polyphenols reduce tumour cell growth and induce apoptosis in both androgen-dependent and androgen-independent prostate cancer cells. J Nutr Biochem. 2008;19:848-855.

Yuanjie Niu et al., Tissue prostate specific antigen (PSA) facilitates refractory prostate tumor progression via enhancing ARA70-regulated androgen receptor trans-activation. Cancer Res. 2008;68;7110-7119.

Zhang J et al., Indole-3-carbinol induces G1 cell cycle arrest and inhibits PSA production in human LNCaP prostate carcinoma cells. Cancer, 2003;98: 2511-2520.

Recommended Reading

Gawler I. *You can conquer cancer*. Michelle Anderson Publishing Pty Ltd, 2001.

Hassed C. *New frontiers in medicine (Volume 2)*. Michelle Anderson Publishing Pty Ltd, 2009.

Kune, G. *The home health guide to a cancer-free family*. Michelle Anderson Publishing Pty Ltd, 2007.

Localised Prostate *Cancer: a guide for men and their families*. Cancer Council of Australia, 2006.

Moyad M. *Promoting wellness for prostate cancer patients*. Ann Arbor Media Group, 2009.

Myers C. *Eating Your Way to better Health: The Prostate Forum Nutrition Guide*. Rivanna Health Publications, Virginia, 2000.

Myers C. *Beating Prostate Cancer: Hormonal Therapy and Diet*. Rivanna Health Publications, Virginia, 2007.

Ornish D. *The Spectrum: A scientifically proven program to feel better, live longer, lose weight and gain health*. Barnes and Noble, 2007.

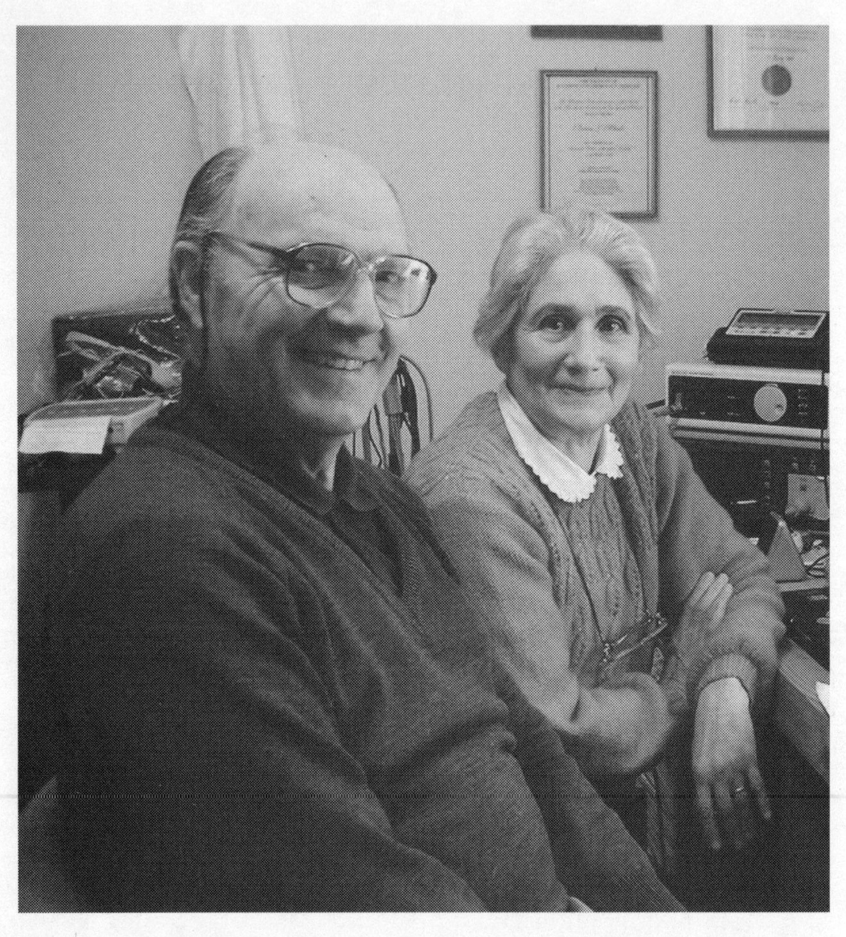

The author Brian Meade and his wife Elizabeth

Notes

Notes